YOGA AND
REHABILITATION

GW00778346

YOGA AND
REHABILITATION

Nilima Patel
B Physiotherapy
PG Diploma in Clinical and Community Psychology
Yoga Certificate Course (YCC)
Yoga Teacher Training Course (YTTC)
Member of Indian Association of Physiotherapy
Senior Faculty at College of Physiotherapy
SSG Hospital and Medical College
Faculty of Medicine
Baroda, Gujarat
India

JAYPEE BROTHERS MEDICAL PUBLISHERS (P) LTD.

New Delhi • Ahmedabad • Bengaluru • Chennai
Hyderabad • Kochi • Kolkata • Lucknow • Mumbai • Nagpur

Published by

Jitendar P Vij
Jaypee Brothers Medical Publishers (P) Ltd
B-3 EMCA House, 23/23B Ansari Road, Daryaganj
New Delhi 110 002, India
Phones: +91-11-23272143, +91-11-23272703, +91-11-23282021, +91-11-23245672,
Rel: +91-11-32558559, Fax: +91-11-23276490, +91-11-23245683
e-mail: jaypee@jaypeebrothers.com   Visit our website: www.jaypeebrothers.com

Branches

- 2/B, Akruti Society, Jodhpur Gam Road Satellite
  Ahmedabad 380 015, Phones: +91-79-26926233, Rel: +91-79-32988717
  Fax: +91-079-26927094 e-mail: ahmedabad@jaypeebrothers.com

- 202 Batavia Chambers, 8 Kumara Krupa Road, Kumara Park East
  Bengaluru 560 001, Phones: +91-80-22285971, +91-80-22382956
  Rel: +91-80-32714073, Fax: +91-80-22281761 e-mail: bangalore@jaypeebrothers.com

- 282 IIIrd Floor, Khaleel Shirazi Estate, Fountain Plaza, Pantheon Road
  Chennai 600 008, Phones: +91-44-28193265, +91-44-28194897
  Rel: +91-44-32972089, Fax: +91-44-28193231 e-mail: chennai@jaypeebrothers.com

- 4-2-1067/1-3, 1st Floor, Balaji Building, Ramkote Cross Road
  Hyderabad 500 095, Phones: +91-40-66610020, +91-40-24758498
  Rel:+91-40-32940929, Fax:+91-40-24758499 e-mail: hyderabad@jaypeebrothers.com

- No. 41/3098, B & B1, Kuruvi Building, St. Vincent Road
  Kochi 682 018, Kerala, Phones: 0484-4036109, +91-0484-2395739,
  +91-0484-2395740 e-mail: kochi@jaypeebrothers.com

- 1-A Indian Mirror Street, Wellington Square
  Kolkata 700 013, Phones: +91-33-22651926, +91-33-22276404, +91-33-22276415
  Rel: +91-33-32901926, Fax: +91-33-22656075 e-mail: kolkata@jaypeebrothers.com

- Lekhraj Market III, B-2, Sector-4, Faizabad Road, Indira Nagar
  Lucknow 226 016   Phones: +91-522-3040553, +91-522-3040554
  e-mail: lucknow@jaypeebrothers.com

- 106 Amit Industrial Estate, 61 Dr SS Rao Road, Near MGM Hospital, Parel
  Mumbai 400 012, Phones: +91-22-24124863, +91-22-24104532
  Rel: +91-22-32926896, Fax: +91-22-24160828 e-mail: mumbai@jaypeebrothers.com

- "KAMALPUSHPA" 38, Reshimbag, Opp. Mohota Science College, Umred Road
  Nagpur 440 009 (MS), Phones: Rel: 3245220, Fax: 0712-2704275
  e-mail: nagpur@jaypeebrothers.com

Yoga and Rehabilitation

© 2008, Nilima Patel

This book has been published in good faith that the material provided by author is original.
Every effort is made to ensure accuracy of material, but the publisher, printer and author
will not be held responsible for any inadvertent error(s). In case of any dispute, all legal
matters are to be settled under Delhi jurisdiction only.

First Edition: **2008**
ISBN 978-81-8448-211-9
Typeset at JPBMP typesetting unit
Printed at Rajkamal Electric Press, B-35/9, G.T. Karnal Road, Delhi-33

To
My Parents
Vimla Patel
and
Sudam Patel

Foreword

In my humble opinion Dr Nilima Sudambhai Patel is a serene, virtuous and God-fearing person. She is quite well known for being a person of high integrity and strong philanthropic attitude towards life. She has done the Yoga Certificate Course and the Yoga Teachers Training Course from the Maharaja Sayajirao Institute of Research in Yog (The Yog Niketan), Baroda. Her exemplary dedication, well defined, disciplined and controlled life, full faith in Yoga and a very deep rooted strong desire to learn it as well as possible, enabled her to understand the intricacies of yoga extremely well. She has learnt about both theoretical and practical aspects of yoga in great detail. At present she has been rendering honorary services as the Teacher of Yoga in the Maharaja Sayajirao Institute of Research in Yoga (The Yoga Niketan), Baroda. She is now an integral part of this institute.

The basic academic discipline of Dr Patel is Physiotherapy and she has been working as the faculty in the College of Physiotherapy, Faculty of Medicine, MS University of Baroda for over 25 years now. When she was the student of YCC and YTTC she conducted many major experiments on the relevance of Yoga to the science of physiotherapy and its application to the medical treatment. She has also worked a lot on the connectivity of yoga and physiotherapy and its usefulness for rehabilitation of patients. This is indeed a unique integration of applied science of yoga and physiotherapy. Her wide experience as a physiotherapist and her deep understanding of yoga have helped her very well to easily assimilate the intricacies and excellence of Yoga and many finer points of physiotherapy. This has resulted in the application of her knowledge of physio-yoga for the betterment of hundreds of her patients and students. This is, I feel, a new and novel approach in the field of physiotherapy and thereby one of the most remarkably welcome features of modern medical treatment. It should prove very good for all concerned. Dr Patel will, I hope, be able to use it further and also guide others too to use it most advantageously in Physiotherapy. As a physiotherapist Dr Patel is very much popular among her patients. She has guided many complicated and challengingly rare cases very successfully and given hope and new life to hundreds of her patients. Her pleasant and graceful looks and her sober, suave, patient understanding and encouraging nature work like elixir for all in general and for her patients in particular.

My heartiest congratulations to Dr Nilima Patel for so successfully connecting yoga and physiotherapy for the welfare of the society. This should be, I feel, considered as her innovation in physiotherapy.

May Goddess "Maa Paraamba" " माँ परंबा " bless her with Her choicest blessings and grant her the desired success in all her efforts to serve humanity. May She bless her with all happiness, peace and prosperity and lead her on the path of religious ways of living a good life.

Dr. Vishnuprasad Acharya
Director
Maharaja Sayajirao Institute of
Research in Yoga (Yoga Niketan)
Baroda

Preface

God Gave You Skill, But Patient's Faith and Confidence
Makes You Great

— A Quotable Quote

Each and every person is unique with his individual way of thinking, emotions, feelings, perception, habits, likes and dislikes.

The human being is a powerhouse, and a constant generator of energy. Only what is required, is to understand its source. I do also believe that the source is the "Self." Self-awareness and self-care have very important role to play in every rehabilitation programme.

Yoga is the journey and destination to the "Self" and rehabilitation is to restore the abilities through the "Self".

Born to Theosophist parents who always imbibed in us that,
  "There is no religion higher than Truth"
  "Healthy Mind leads to a healthy Body"
  "Service to Mankind is service to God",
I always used to contemplate a lot on these aspects of their thinking.

I also believe that a good physiotherapist has to be first a good psychologist, and always made an effort to educate my students on this aspect. The interest in the field of psychology and results on power of mind encouraged me to do a Postgraduate Diploma course in Clinical and Community Psychology. But still I felt something essential was missing—The knowledge and experience about the "Self".

I realized that higher than hands, heart and mind is our soul (Self). In search of "Self" for which I climbed the stairs of many spiritual centers of Abode and faith like Brahmakumaris at Mount

Abu, where I experienced the "silencing of mind" through Rajyoga meditation, Theosophical Society at Adyar which encourgaed me to follow the path of truth, Ramkrishna Mission at Kanyakumari, where Swami Vivekanand's concept of "Truth and Fearlessness" inspired me, Arbindo ashram at Pondicherry where I understood the meaning of "selfless service" and pilgrimage places of Amarnath, Kedarnath, Badrinath, Gangotri, Yamnotri, Rameshwaram and many more. All this lead to realization of "an invisible guiding force."

Eventually, I also climbed the stairs of Maharaja Sayajirao Institute of Research in Yoga—Yogniketan, Baroda, where I studied, analyzed, contemplated and practiced Bhagwan Patanjali's Ashtang yoga and Yogsutras. I realized that "Everything is within me" Gyana (knowledge), Bhakti (devotion) and Karma (action)—"The source of powerhouse." Sri Sri Ravishankarji's Sudarshan Kriya practice strengthened my belief in the concept of Prana and Pranayama.

Although yoga is found in association with religious belief and practices, it is itself a religion. It is essentially a process, a teaching, a method and may be practiced equally either within or outside a religious system. It is based on laws of nature whose applications have been established by experiment and may be felt by experience.

I experienced myself that if the habitual tendencies of mind to react to external stimuli can be regulated (so that it can become quiet) to achieve calm, the mind will be as clear as the still water of a lake reflecting the "Self".

The measure of this "Self" is **Spiritual Quotient**, which is an integration of *Intelligence, Emotional and Moral Quotient*. It connects human being through interaction and with feelings of respect and regard for each other. It is self-awareness and self-motivation dimension for rehabilitation.

In the times of great medical advancement and research, the philosophical, psychological, metaphysical, spiritual basis of yoga may be accepted or denied, partially or completely, but my experience with this enriching yogic practice made me to believe that although not an alternative therapy yet there can be no greater rehabilitation method for disease prevention and cure than that achieved by yogic practices.

Yoga and rehabilitation is based on the principles of Ashtangyoga and its application for prevention and management of many psychosomatic disorders. According to me, this practical, economical, spiritual and most prestigious approach is aimed at refining and enriching the consciousness of people based on which psychophysical health, energy and rehabilitation can be achieved.

The two sections in this book are concerned with:

(a) Principles and psychophysical aspects of different types of yoga disciplines, mainly the Ashtangyoga and the difference between the physical and yogic exercise and also about **physio-yoga**, the integrated approach in rehabilitation.

(b) Application of this integrated approach in rehabilitation, in respiratory, cardiovascular, neuromuscular, musculoskeletal and women's issues related disorders, based on principles of biomechanics and exercise therapy.

In writing this book, my effort has been to offer everyone, the "Role of Self" in Rehabilitation. The book is for all persons associated with rehabilitation—the patient, the family, the community, the students and the experts. It is a new concept, which I believe, needs to be experienced and felt.

Emotional calm aids in getting rid of negativity and acquire relaxation, stability and balanced state, which strengthen the stress coping mechanism, mental and physical and immunity for complete health and rehabilitation.

To define in one line, the book is about restoring complete health (mental, physical, social, spiritual) by realizing the "Self" (through yoga).

Nilima Patel

The Words from Within

In a normal cultured and civlized society, man can never work in isolation. It is not a matter of simple social interdependency about which I am talking here, it is something much more than this and something quite different that I am referring to here. In all efforts and achievements of man, there are always some sources of direct or indirect contributions. Over the last decade that I have spent evolving "**Physio-yoga**: An Integrated Approach of Physiotherapy and Yoga in Rehabilitation", I have realized a humbling truth that my pleasure in writing, it has been enhanced by the vision, faith, belief, confidence, understanding, encouragement, inspiration, guidance, advice, help, comments, etc. received from my teachers, idols, superiors, colleagues, dear and near ones and many well wishers. It would be, thereof, very ungrateful of me, if I do not acknowledge them (contributions) here with a sense of gratitude.

First of all I express my genuine gratefulness to my teachers who guided me through the path of self-belief, honesty, sincerity, selfless service and the consequent hard work and discipline.

It was my school teacher, US Cholkar Sir who strongly believed that I showed an apititude for science and hence, insisted that I should join the science stream in higher secondary education. He advised me to study science and later join the fine and noble profession of physiotherapy. Cholkar Sir's belief and confidence in me, thus, made me that I am today. I am immensely thankful to him for his interest, advice and guidance.

Next I owe my heartiest thanks to Late Dr. John Gohel, Ex-Head, Department of Physiotherapy, Faculty of Medicine, MS University of Baroda, who always freely expressed his belief and confidence in my potentiality as a student earlier and later on as a colleague. He instilled self-belief in me which guides me even today. Had he been with us today, he would have been very proud to see this book and also very happy to mark me as someone who has tried to justify his vision. I gratefully seek Late Dr. John Gohel Sir's blessings from above.

My Yoga Guru Shri Vishnuprasad Acharyaji at the Yoga Niketan, Baroda had a fine faith in me. He encouragingly asked me to spread the message of yoga as a scientifically disciplined method of training body, mind and soul that inculcates a disciplined and controlled life following the Vedic ways and wisdom. I feel no hestitation to state here that **physio-yoga** is the result of Acharyaji's inspiration and faith in me. I acknowledge my depth of gratitude to him from the bottom of my heart.

Dr Kiran Singhlot, my Guru at the Yoga Niketan, Baroda, taught me the techniques of yoga and the principles of yoga and Pranayama excellently making the difficult points very easy to understand and the complex principles so simple to follow that it became very easy to learn and follow yoga in daily practice. He used to excite and instruct the intellect of his students quite inovatively! What an experience it was to learn yoga from Dr Singhlot!! I very sincerely thank him for teaching me yoga so well and so easefully and interestingly.

I have always derived inspiration from my professional idol or role model madam Daulat Dastoor. Her nature, professional creative attitude and the fine way of working have always inspired me to work to the best of my ability and to develop a good creative attitude towards my profession. Madam Dastoor always inspires me to do better than before and always improves upon my worth. I clearly owe a deep sense of gratitude to Dastoor Madam for all this.

Our school teacher, BG Bhatt Sir instilled a good sense of discipline into us. He was a strict disciplinarian and always said that discipline should guide us in our day-to-day life. This early lesson of discipline helped me easily understand and accept that yoga is something quite in the line of discipline of body, mind and soul. My thanks to BG Bhatt Sir.

My special thanks are reserved for my nine-year-old friend. Ayush. Chiranjeeva Ayush has been an inexplicable source of challenge and motivation to me professionally. While guiding him, my professional knowledge, skills, abilities and efficiency were at test and he helped me a lot to do my best for him with his remarkable courage and brave attitude towards life. His enthusiastic and dignified promise that he would buy a copy of my book has greatly enthused me too personally. Thank you Ayush!

It would be very ungrateful of me, if I do not express my deep sense of gratefulness to my present Dean Dr Kamal Pathak, Dr Pathak always asked me to do something concrete in my field. In many meetings of ours he talked, discussed and even argued with me encouragingly to do something new, something different, something useful in the field of physiotherapy using my interests, abilities and innovative nature in the best possible ways. I thankfully acknowledge this indirect contribution from Dr Pathak.

I sincerely wish to place on record my thanks to the Organizing Committee of the 44th Annual Conference of Indian Association of Physiotherapists at Ahmedabad. I was gracefully invited by them to give a talk on **My Experience with Yoga** in a symposium. It was at this symposium that the seeds of writing this book were sown.

My niece Chiranjeeva Janhavi, a journalist today, made some very useful suggestions regarding how to make this book interesting even for young readers. She also initially taught me how to use computer. My heartiest thanks to Chiranjeeva Janhavi.

How can I ever fail to thankfully take on record the immense help I have received from my youngest sister Anjana and my brother-in-law Ramakant. The process of writing this book with computer graphics, sketches, drawings, labeling and layout would have never been completed without their fine work. Very painstakingly they entered into computer every last bit of research, new ideas and thoughts and meticulously created order in the deluge of information. They did this work as "labour of love". Every bit of labour was done very enthusiastically without any feeling of boredom or fatigue! I very genuinely acknowledge my debt of gratitude to these two dear ones of mine.

My little niece and nephew Anushka and Tanay have also obliged me by sacrificing their parents' attention and care for them when they were busy with the computer work of this book. Both little ones let go their time of care and cuddling to make their parents free to work incessantly to complete my work in a very short duration of just four months. I feel extremely thankful to these two little ones.

Mr. Abhijit Bose, very nicely informed me about the initiative taking policy to give platform to authors who are interested in sharing their thoughts and views with people on different branches of knowledge in Medical Sciences. I am immensely thankful to him.

I thank M/s Jaypee Brothers Medical Publishers not only for publishing this book but also for displaying a good deal of consideration and courage in introducing an absoultely new concept of **physio-yoga**. They are actually, it is well known, the renowned publishers of books on Medical Sciences. This time, they have taken, it seems, an exception to their rule.

I owe my sincere thanks to my friends Dr Jayshree Mehta (Vice Chancellor, Sumandeep University), Rina, Gita Siddharth, Trupti and Dr D.C. Master (Professor in Anatomy, Faculty of Medicine, M.S. University) for their constant feedbacks and suggestions before and during the process of writing this book. Also I thank my colleagues at the Medical College and the yoga teachers, trainers and disciples at the Yog Niketan, Baroda for their suggestions to me to contribute something to the society by putting in black and white my thoughts and ideas on physio-yoga.

Had my family's interest, untiring and wonderful support and every encouraging attitude not been there constantly throughout the process of my growth and development little or nothing would have been possible for me to do in life. I have, therefore, always felt immensely grateful to my family for the ever-supportive kindness. I end here with my father's words always that "God is Great."

PHOTO CREDIT BY ALOK BRAHMABHATT OF JANHAVI PATEL. MY HEARTIEST BLESSINGS TO BOTH THESE YOUNG ONES.

Contents

Section 1

Chapter 1

MY EXPERIENCE WITH YOGA

"A Yogi believes that his body has been given to him by the Lord not for the enjoyment alone, but also for the service of his fellowmen, during wakeful moment of his life."

— A quotable quote.

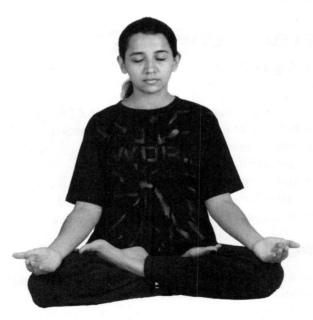

Fig. 1.1: Padmasana (The lotus posture)

"Experience is the best teacher."This statement I recollect was taught to me by one of my Gurus – teachers while I was in school. Moreover he always said to me after I became a teacher that, "Learning is a continuous process and one is student for all his lifetime." These two aspects of being a student for a lifetime, and learning through experience have inspired me to share my experiences with Yoga.

I have been in the profession of Physiotherapy since last twenty-five years. I always used to think and speak high about the modalities used for therapeutic purpose in different areas of Physiotherapy applications. No doubt, I am proud to be a physiotherapist, but after studying, learning experiencing and feeling about Yoga Science, I believe I am blessed to be a Yoga student. The student in me of physiotherapy is enriched by my experience with Yoga Science and its application as one of the Adjunct Therapy in almost all "Self created Disorders."

YOGA EDUCATED ME...

What Yoga is Not ...

- It is not a form or *type of exercise*.
- It is not *a gymnastic exercise* or an acrobatic skill.
- It is not *an alternative therapy* for any disease control or cure.
- It is not to be *experimented* and *proved*.
- It is not a *philosophy or doctrine*.
- It is not *escapism* from facing reality of life.
- It is not *penance* as always misunderstood.
- It is not to *gain mystical powers* and *miraculous achievements*.

But Yoga Is ...

- It is a special form of Physical Exercise through mind control.
- It is the path, that teaches one to believe in *Self* and live life with positivism, peace and perfection.

- It is an Adjunct Therapy, a supportive therapy to heal the mind and body.
- It is to be experienced and felt.
- It is one of the six orthodox systems of Indian Philosophy.
- It is a methodical, sincere and honest practice of its disciplines.
- It *prescribes penance* and *not punishment* for the wrong done.
- It is a *spiritual endeavor*.
- It is to gain *supreme harmonization* of body, mind and soul.
- It is the *mean and measure to achieve* Positive Health.

YOGA ENLIGHTENED IN ME ...

- The knowledge of *Prana* and the great powers of *Prana*.
- The Prana that moves the universe is *Cosmic Prana*.
- The *minute atom* to the *biggest solar system* is the result of Cosmic Prana.
- The finest manifestation of *Vibrating Prana* is the *mind.*
- It is vital *source of energy* that exists everywhere.
- The Prana is the cause of *heat, light, motion* and *electricity.*
- It is also the cause of our *will power* and the manifestation of each soul.
- The diaphragm which *contracts* and *relaxes* because of some nervous energy is due to Prana.
- This Prana is located in spinal column from which *motor* and *sensory nerves* branch out and spread all over the organs.
- The *activity of heart* is also regulated by this energy.
- The centres that generate the energy are located in spinal column – *The Chakras* (Nervous Plexus).
- The *power of Prana* is also the cause of all *mental functions.*
- This *Prana* exists in air, water and food, hence, the concept is of sensible living, drinking and eating.

- The entire *respiratory* system functions on the power of *Prana*.
- Enslaved by desires and materialistic gain, we gradually weaken this Prana and loose the *power to conserve* its energy.
- To *develop* thinking power, will power and intellectual faculties, we must learn the method of *conserving this nervous energy*.

"Yogic practice is to know this prana, understand its mechanism and strengthen its function on which, I also believe our auto-immune system functions."

YOGA EMPOWERED IN ME ...

- *The Thought* of "Belief in Self" Our past experiences, sanskars, company, friends and our attitude are responsible for our stability and peace in life.
- *The Core Values* of "Knowledge, Purity (thought, speech and action), Love for all, Peace in life, Happiness in life, Will power and Compassion." To empower the mind is to empower all values. Empowering thoughts and values create empowering beliefs and empowered confidence.
- *The Attitude* of "Humility"—which is very close to Karmayoga philosophy. One who is humble achieves longevity, knowledge and goodness.
- *The Virtues* of "Dedication" which motivated me to perform my role in life with a sense of duty and as an offering to Lord without any rewards and attachment.

Virtue: Dedication : "Do good and forget."

- *The Approach* of "Spiritual Tool"—The power of Self in the management programme of a patient's education and guidance so as to prevent the re-occurrence of many Functional disorders. Self-realization improves receptivity of the subconscious mind, channelizes the thoughts towards optimism, strengthens willpower and recuperates the nerve centres to flow energy to heal faster and better.

YOGA ENCOURAGED ME ...

- *To grow everyday*, with my patients and learn from them. It is because of their faith in me that today I am able to share this experience with everyone (Change is inevitable, growth is optional).
- *To convey whatever I realized through Self-introspection*. It made me aware of the fact, that instead of hunting for the disabilities in a patient, I should make an effort to find out the abilities left in him, and strengthen those abilities to take over the function of the lost ones, so that he can once again live with confidence and dignity, as an integral part of family and society.
- *To understand* the fact that, to mould someone's attitude is more important than changing his physique (Healing the mind heals the body).
- *To implement* "relaxation postures, regulated breathing techniques and free, frank conversation" with all the patients and their family members irrespective of whatever disorder or dysfunction they have come with. Empathetic communication lessens the pain significantly and improves the acceptance and tolerance level.
- *To harness* "patient's energy" and *prevent* it from being wasted "in tension", so that they can participate with enthusiasm in the **Rehabilitation programme**.

YOGA ENRICHED ME ...

- With the *knowledge* that "Air is food". It is the most essential food and one should seek to breathe air at the highest nutritional value, which means highly charged with *Prana* or life force. The most vitalising air, they say is by the sea, mountains, lakes and large open spaces.

- With the *knowledge* of "Sensible eating". One should always eat as per the hunger (physiological need) and not as per the appetite (desire). Moderation in eating is very important for Positive health.

- With this *"Value based Approach"- Integrated Approach*, that considers Spiritual quotient (Self) the foundation of total healing process. Spiritual Quotient is integration of Intelligence Quotient, Moral Quotient and Emotional Quotient. When Intelligence and Moral Quotient of the healer gets tuned with the Emotional Quotient of a patient; the result of it, speaks for itself. Spiritual Quotient connects human beings through interaction with respect and regards for each other. This is a Self-motivated dimension.

My experince with Yoga is nurturing and nourishing me everyday. It has made my life more content and purposefully growthful.

The contents of all the chapters are penned down based on what I have studied, felt and experienced during these years, with the inspirational books that I referred and the Yogic guidance given to me, by my Guru's in the learning process.

Much is to be said and more is to be done, but the most of it needs to be practised in my approach towards the rehabilitation process. It is rightly said:

"Charity begins at home."

"Practise before you preach."

Chapter 2   YOGA TO ME IS ...

"You need not have a face which makes you look in the mirror often, but have such a face which makes people look at you often."

— A quotable quote.

Yoga is to make one healthy of body, clear and balanced of mind and stable of emotions. Most of us are not aware of the qualities we possess, the abilities we have, and seek the strength from outside. Hence a *transformational change is necessary*. Yoga helps in making us aware of our powers and skill.

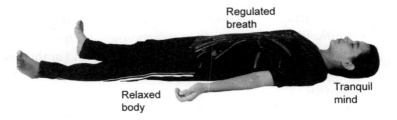

Regulated breath

Relaxed body

Tranquil mind

Fig. 2.1: Shavasana (The corpse posture)

YOGA TO ME IS...

1. *"Yoga Karmesu Kaushalam": Bhagwad Gita*
   "Work is worship." As per the knowledge of Bhagwad Gita, whatever work one does, it should be done with *devotion, dedication and determination.* The work should be performed with positivity, zeal, efficiency and with a pleasant, cheerful, selfless attitude. A feeling of contentment and happiness is experienced as its result.

   "Yoga is skill in work and efficiency in its performance."

2. *"Samatwam Yoga Uchhyate": Bhagwad Gita.*
   - *Attachment* to materialistic things and desire for material gains is the main cause of our sorrow and misery. *It is due to ignorance.*
   - This *ignorance* gives rise to *feelings of pain and pleasure, likes and dislikes, hope and despair, depression and elation.*
   - These feelings create *emotional turmoil* and disturb the mind, which *affect the stability and harmony of body,* leading to all ailments and sufferings.
   - Yoga *tranquilizes the mind, regulates the thoughts* and *calms the emotions* thereby harmonizing the body in all situations.

   "Yoga is supreme harmonization of mind and body."

3. *"Yoga Chittavritti Nirodh": Bhagwan Patanjali.*
   - *Chitta* is the mind stuff in psychology. *Vrittis* are the thought waves, which give rise to feelings and emotions as a function of the subconscious mind. *Nirodh* is to control.
   - Yoga philosophy teaches us that mind is not *"Intelligence and Consciousness."* It has only a borrowed intelligence. The "Atman" is intelligence itself, is pure consciousness. *The mind merely reflects that consciousness and so appears to be conscious.*

- Yoga is to *control the disturbing thought* waves and discipline the mind and know the true nature of the "Real Self." Realization of the egolessness state of consciousness is the Absolute Resolution of Yoga.

"Yoga is the control of thought waves in the mind."

MY PERCEPTION OF ASHTANG YOGA LADDER

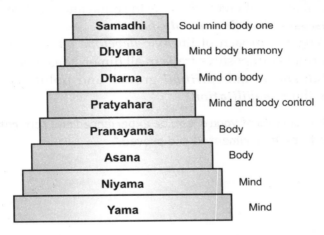

Samadhi	Soul mind body one
Dhyana	Mind body harmony
Dharna	Mind on body
Pratyahara	Mind and body control
Pranayama	Body
Asana	Body
Niyama	Mind
Yama	Mind

Fig. 2.2: The Rajyoga ladder—The eight limbs

- Yoga inculcates moral values in an individual. The first two steps of Rajyoga ladder, *Yama* (social discipline) and *Niyama* (individual discipline) signify the code of conduct of one's life patterns. One who is adjusted to surrounding is adjusted to one's own self (*Yama*) and one who is in harmony with his own self, harmonizes with each and every person, situation and events around him (*Niyama*). Yama and Niyama are the result of a serene mind. A regulated controlled mind is the foundation of one's *pleasant personality*.
- The next two steps of *Asana* (the lubricant of psychosomatic machine-body) and *Pranayama* (the

vacuum cleaner of psychosomatic machine) *regulate, replenish and rejuvenate* the body. A stable erect posture with a regulated breath leads to a *striking personality*.

- The fifth step, *Pratyahara* (withdrawal from senses) controls the mind and the body, whereas the sixth step *Dharna* (concentration) improves the balance and harmony between mind and body. The seventh step of *Dhyana* (meditation) *strengthens* the stress coping mechanism, thereby *liberating* the mind and the body from *diseases, disorders and dysfunctions*.

The Yogic approach of lifestyle *develops and matures* an individual with positive traits in all dimensions of *physical, mental, social and spiritual* growth and upliftment and hence the *Rehabilitation*.

"Achievements of yoga are to be experienced and felt, rather than to be experimented and proved."

Chapter 3

YOGA TO ME
AS A
PHYSIOTHERAPIST

"Healing depends on the qualities of the healer. Medical practitioners continuously transfer their specific vibrations to their patients. This is the healing touch, a result of inner tranquility."

So much is said about Body Mind and Soul, today. This is the triology of human endowment. To improve the mind without cultivation of our physical gift would be a very hollow victory. Elevating our mind and body to our highest level without nurturing the soul would leave us feeling very empty and unfulfilled. But when we dedicate our energies to unlocking the full potential of all three of our human endowments, we will taste the power of Positive Health, Comprising of Physical, Mental, Social and Spiritual Dimensions.

A physiotherapist first needs to be a good psychologist. Physiotherapy and Psychology both have their origins in Yoga Discipline, more than three thousand years ago.

"Physiotherapy is the means, Yoga is the path."

YOGA: A PSYCHOLOGIST'S PERSPECTIVE

"Healthy mind leads to healthy body"

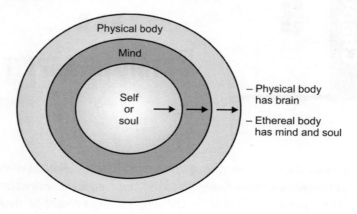

Fig. 3.1: Journey within → without path

All source of knowledge is within us and all source of power is also within us. It is only a matter of understanding our inner potential. The journey within - to - without (Fig. 3.1) leads us through the path to reach the destination of Positive Health.

Let us understand these three components of Self (Soul), Mind (Psyche) and Body (Physique).

The Self

- It is Reality within each individual.
- It is above mind and part of the Absolute.
- It helps in living in the Present with Positivity and Persistence.
- It helps us to sow seeds of Creativity and Happiness.
- It cultivates empowering thoughts in the Mind.
- It is the self that needs to be enlightened for Positive Health.

- It is the transformation of this "Inner Self" to the Outer Existence that can prevent and eliminate any disease, dysorder and dysfunction.

The Mind

- It is that which Thinks, Feels, Believes and Imagines.
- It is the "seat" or "subject" of Consciousness.
- It is Omnipresent and exists in everything that we can perceive or cannot see or conceptualize, states the ancient wisdom.
- It is the higher form of energy and function of the Brain.
- It perceives, analyses, integrates and interprets Stimuli.
- It strengthens the receptivity and perception of the Subconscious mind, which leads to Positive Health.

The Physical Body

- It is the crudest manifestation of human being.
- It is lowest in scale, although very necessary.
- It houses the "Self".
- It is important for the human being for his growth in his present state of development.
- It is the Holy Temple where the Soul resides.
- It is this body, which needs to be kept in good and positive shape and state, with vibrance and vigor, as unhealthy body cannot obey mind's orders effectively.

"Journey and destination to the Self is Yoga"

YOGA: THE PHYSIOTHERAPIST'S PERSPECTIVE

"Healthy body nurtures a healthy mind"

Yoga is not to stand on one's head (Shirsasana) but it is instead to stand firmly on one's feet and face life with all its pressures and problems, stresses (mental and physical) and tensions (emotional and muscular) with courage, consistency and compatibility (Fig. 4.1).

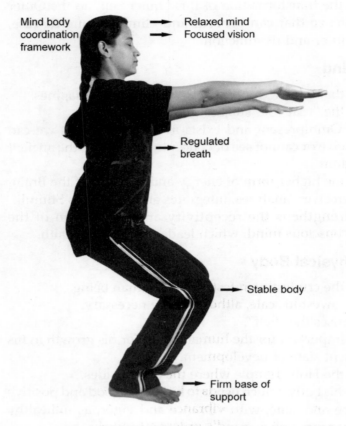

Mind body coordination framework

Relaxed mind
Focused vision

Regulated breath

Stable body

Firm base of support

Fig. 3.2: Modified Uttkatasana—A balanced posture

A Physiotherapist with:

Vision – to understand and assess the patient's problems

Values – to educate and guide the patient with positivity

Mission – to heal,

can be a conceptual bridge between the mind and the body, with a Yogic Therapeutic Approach for Prevention and Elimination of any Disease, Disorder or Dysfunction.

The need is a simple, practical, economic, non-invasive, subjective, self-prescriptive tool "THE SELF" with

- The Spiritual Core of Assessment: Empathetic Listening.
- The Spiritual Approach of Management: Interpathic Guidelines.

A physiotherapist's ultimate goal is Energy Conservation and Functional Rehabilitation with the concept of Erect Posture, Breath Regulation, along with WILL, Discipline and Determination towards the path of early recovery and rehabilitation.

"Body is the holy temple where the Soul resides."

THE YOGIC SCIENCE IN PHYSIOTHERAPY

Yoga is a science in itself, which needs no proof and experiments. It is suited to prevent physical and mental illnesses and to protect the body, generally developing an inevitable sense of self-reliance and assurance.

The physical approach with Exercise-therapy, Electrotherapy Modalities and Manipulation techniques may treat a patient but along with this, the Spiritual Approach of Yoga will heal the patient.

Stress (Mental and Physical) leading to Pain, Disability, Misinformation and Fear has been spreading like an epidemic today and showing no sign of abating inspite of advancement in research and technology in Modern medicine and Therapies. Tension is a Universal problem today. It could be mental, muscular or total.

Emotions, Thoughts, Feelings, Beliefs, Behaviour, Personality, Lifestyle, Aging process, Occupation and other innumerable traits are responsible in causing *Psychosomatic Disorders.*

The word *"Psychosomatic"* is widely misunderstood to describe an imaginary disorder experienced by people who are mentally abnormal or an exaggeration of symptoms that are structurally based. To set the record straight, psychosomatic symptoms are real, they occur in normal people and are universal.

These mind – body symptoms exist to serve a purpose. If you thwart that purpose by taking away the symptom without dealing with its cause, then the brain will find a substitute symptom or disorder in form of a physical illness.

"Healing the mind heals the body and training the mind trains the body."

PHYSIO-YOGA

Majority of patients attending any physiotherapy set-up for therapy, are having disorders with a Psychosomatic origin, may it be in a field of Musculoskeletal Physiotherapy (Pain Syndrome), Neuromuscular Physiotherapy (CV Strokes, Parkinson's Syndromes), Cardiovascular Physiotherapy (Hypertension and Cardiac Conditions), Respiratory Physiotherapy (Bronchial Asthma, Restrictive Pulmonary diseases), Biomechanics and Exercise Therapy (Postural problems). Almost all these disturbances are as a result of deficient or poor stress coping mechanisms and lowered immunity.

Self-realization is the main aim of Yoga. This Realized Self enhances the recovery from any illness and dysfunction, by acceptance and perception of the ailment with positivity.

1. *The Analgesic Effect of Yoga* (Asanas and Pranayama), through the Central mechanism of Paingate Control Theory and due to the balance between Peripheral Nervous system and Autonomic Nervous system, helps in alleviating and preventing many painful syndromes.

2. *The Motor Recovery Effect of Yoga* (Asanas, Pranayama and Pratyahara), hastens motor recovery, improves neurological mechanisms, i.e. Postural mechanisms by neural conditioning enhancing the functional recovery in Neurological disorders.

3. *The Tranquilising Effect of Yoga* (Pranayama and Meditation) sedates the mind, strengthens the stress coping mechanism, and improves immunity, thereby overcoming and relieving Cardiovascular disorders.

4. *The Immunoenhancing Effect of Yoga* (Asana, Pranayama and Meditation) activates the Reticulo–Endothilial System, thereby increasing body's resistance to disease, preventing complications and enhancing recovery from Respiratory disorders.

5. *The Homeostatic Effect of Yoga* (The Raj Yoga – Ashtang Yoga ladder of eight steps—Yama, Niyama, Asana, Pranayama, Pratyahara, Dharna, Dhyana and Samadhi) regulates and harmonises the Nervous system and the Endocrine glands, thereby enhancing the stress coping mechanisms and accelerates recovery and relief in Metabolic disorder.

CONCLUSIONS

- A heart full of love, a mind full of vision and hands full of skills is the true nature of a healer.
- All three dimensions of Soul, Mind and Body are necessary to achieve the discreet goal of Positive Health.
- Healing and Relief should be by thoughts and action.
- Interpathy strengthens an individual's immune system and heals thoroughly and gives long lasting effect.
- Yoga is not a substitute for any physiotherapy modality or clinical skill, but it can enable a more Integrated Approach in Rehabilitation through Positive Health. (Physical, Mental, Social and Spiritual).
- Physiotherapy—The Yogic Way, will awaken the physical potential and lead the patient to live with a strong dynamic existence.

Chapter 4

YOGA IN HEALTH CARE

"Spirituality is the art of using our inner resources of peace, love, positivity and compassion for the benefit and healing of ourselves and others."

YOGA IS HEALTH PRESERVER AND HEALTH PROMOTER

- The importance and realization of MIND BODY CONCEPT is once again emerging as a powerful effective *means of 'Healing' rather than 'Therapy'* in its own sense and with its own potentials and limitations.

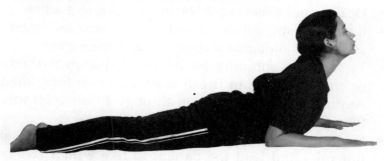

Fig. 4.1: Bhujangasana (The cobra posture)

- Yoga eliminates *"Compassion Fatigue"* and illuminates **spiritual dimensions** in Health Care Approaches. It is an experienced science that applies *"Spirituality – The Missing Dimension"* in the management programme of all Psychosomatic disorders.

- Yoga is *Telepathic connections* of the healer with the patient, having an *Empathetic outlook* and following *Interpathic Guidelines* in healing approaches rather than *Sympathetic Attitudes* which could weaken the morale of the patient.

- Yoga is a *Self Prescription and Self Management* guideline for those who have to lead others and those who want to follow these guidelines through times of accelerating change.

"Yoga is simple, safe, effective and a highly economic form of adjunctive therapy."

HEALTH CARE PROFESSIONALS ARE SAID TO BE MESSENGERS OF GOD

- *Ishwara* (God) in Yoga is *Omnipresent, Omnipotent and Omniscient* who leads to complete *self control, freedom from illness, physical fitness, cheerfulness, hope, confidence and bliss.*

- The Yogic Approach of Healing brings sparkle in patient's life and spreads light all over with positivity, serenity and *strengthens their immune system.*

- *Spiritual Approach* in Health Care Management depends on *core values of Love, Care, Compassion, Competence, Confidentiality, Integrity, Responsibility, Advocacy and Spirit of Inquiry of the Healer.* This approach inculcates sobriety, simplicity, humility, humbleness and a feeling of belongingness and togetherness in patient's management. *This gives the patient a renewal sense of purpose in life.*

"An act becomes beneficial if the intention is to benefit others."

ULTIMATE GOAL OF YOGA IS ENERGY CONSERVATION

- Yoga is to change one's potential energy into kinetic energy physically, mentally, socially and spiritually, as the *ultimate goal of Yoga is Energy Conservation.*
- Yoga helps in *strengthening receptivity of the subconscious mind,* thereby achieving harmony between mind and body which results in prevention and elimination of all psychosomatic disorders.
- Health consciousness is increasing these days more than awareness. *Yogic exercises are unrivalled as they are Preventive as well as Curative with its purpose of total relaxation at all levels.*
- Just as science of medicine has four divisions, i.e. *disease, cause of disease, medicine and recovery so* also Yoga philosophy has four divisions.
  Samsara (life), *cause of Samsara* (cause of living), *means of release* (means of liberation), *release* (liberation).

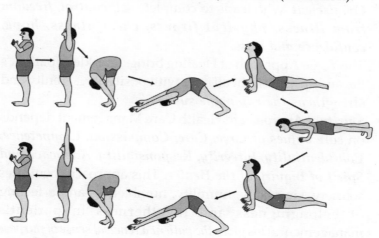

Fig. 4.2: The Sun Salutation Cycle
The human potential energy converted into the kinetic energy

There are many variations and interpretations of the *Suryanamaskar* (Sun salutatin cycle). This is one of them.

- A man with a sound mind and perfect health is the king of whole world once he understands these four divisions. His sound health depends on appropriate balance of food, air, water, regular exercise and mental and social discipline to channelise and harmonize him.

"Yoga is the means and the path to sound health"

5 PATHS OF YOGA

"The Yogi is superior to the performer of penance. (Bhakti). He is also deemed superior to those who have attained True Knowledge (Gyana). He is considered greater than the performer of actions (Karma) as per the scriptures. Therefore Arjuna, follow the path of a Yogi."

— Bhagwad Gita (VI-46)

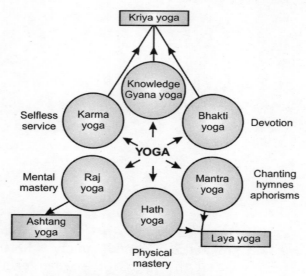

Fig. 5.1: Classification of Paths of Yoga

YOGA IN PHILOSOPHY

- The ancient saints used *Yoga* as a means to explore the exterior and the interior world and ultimately achieved the knowledge and wisdom of *Vedas, Upanishads* and *Shastras*, which have been passed down to the world.
- The Classical Indian Philosophy is divided into six schools called the "*Shad Darshan.*" Shad means six and *Darshan* means to see, or the mirror to see the soul. All six schools are the efforts of many *Rishis* and Intellectuals. They are:

  Kapila's   *SANKHYA*
  Patanjali's   *YOGA*
  Gautama's   *NYAYA SUTRA*
  Kanada's   *VAISHESHIKA*
  Jaimini's   *PURVAMIMAMSA*
  Badrayana's   *UTTARMIMAMSA*
- *Sankhya* specifies that goal of human life is to seek liberation from three kinds of sufferings.
  - Accidental: e.g. earthquake: not in our hands
  - Bodily: e.g. disease: with diagnosis and medicines.
  - Spiritual: e.g. Ignorance: with *darshana* and right knowledge.

  Yoga philosophy is thus about gaining control over oneself and his or her surroundings in order to gain liberation. Right knowledge is supreme means of liberation.

  SANKHYA and YOGA are closely related. Sankhya covers the theoretical part whereas Yoga forms the practical side or Sankhya's practical application.

PATHS OF YOGA

When it comes to classifying and grouping the systems of Yoga, one finds difference of opinion among scholars. The reason for it is that the paths of Yoga overlap and interpenetrate to such an extent that several classifications have validity.

All types of Yoga other than Hatha Yoga are mainly meditative. To name them and to indicate their nature briefly, they are:

1. Bhakti Yoga: Union by love and devotion.

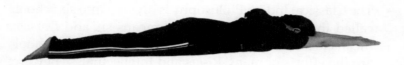

Fig. 5.2: Bhakti–Samarpanasana—The feeling of surrender to God

- It touches the mind and washes out the impurities of the mind.
- It is simple, sweet, gentle and natural.
- An **emotional** man finds his way to the Creator through Love and Devotion.
- It is a genuine search for "Ishwara – God."
- It generates a feeling of total surrender to God.
- A Bhakt (devotee) performs selfless service in name of God.
- This could be the favorite Yoga of Indian masses.
- Its disciplines are those of rites and singing songs of praise in name of the worshipped deity.
- All acts and the food eaten are with a feeling that strength is gained to serve the Lord.
- He, who knows that all creation belongs to the Lord, will not be puffed with pride or drunk with power.
- *Physical power without* Bhakti *is lethal.*
- It may sometimes prove dangerous if followed blindly.
- It may breed communalism and fanaticism if human emotions are not directed properly.

"Bhakti is intense love to God - The way of Emotional Rapport."

2. Karma Yoga: Union by action and service.

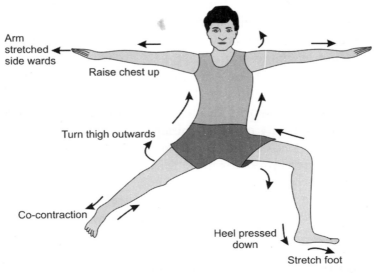

Arm stretched side wards

Raise chest up

Turn thigh outwards

Co-contraction

Heel pressed down

Stretch foot

Fig. 5.3: Karma—Virbhadrasana-II—The way of dedicated work

- *Karma:* Sanskrit word *'Kri'* means 'to do', hence all action "is to work".
- Its main effect is on the body.
- The **Active** man finds realization through work and duty.
- Its philosophy is 'service to mankind is service to God.'
- It is a path of selfless action and service without the thought of fruits and action.
- *Karma* is done with renunciation of all attachments, all feelings of success or failure, gain or loss, victory or defeat, pleasure or pain.
- *Karma* shapes character – Swami Vivekananda.
- *Karma* decides for a man what he deserves and what he can assimilate.
- It motivates a person to be a soldier, always in a battlefield of life, without any desire for applause, name, fame, money and gratitude.

- It leads towards total freedom. Attachment breeds *Moha* (attachment) and *Moha* obstructs right karma (action) and without right action no freedom is possible.
- It upholds the theory of making one's own destiny, as *"action changes fate."*
- The quality of one's life comes down to the quality of one's contribution, i.e. Karma.
- When one works to elevate the life of others, one automatically elevates oneself.
- Noble deeds breed sound and perfect health.
- *Karmayoga* prepares mind for Gyana.

"Karmayoga is wisdom in work or skillful living amongst activities, harmony and moderation." - The way of Dedicated Work.

3. Gyana Yoga: Union by knowledge

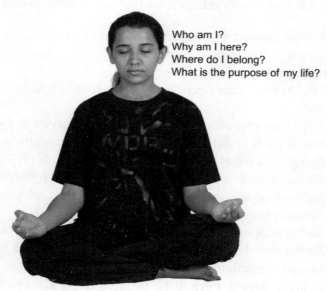

Who am I?
Why am I here?
Where do I belong?
What is the purpose of my life?

Fig. 5.4: Gyana yoga: Sukhasana—Easy posture—The way of wisdom

- Its main effect is on **Soul.**
- The **Intellectual** man finds realization through knowledge.
- It connects one with reality and helps to visualize things in its true sense.
- It is the path of *spiritual knowledge and wisdom.*
- The disciplines of this path are of *study and meditation.*
- Theory of evolution stresses on "survival of the fittest". It is a wise man, who survives through education and knowledge.
- It gives us true nature of our soul, which is omnipresent and omniscient, and has no form or shape.
- The knowledge of *Atman* (Soul) and *Parmatma* (God) destroys ignorance, pain and sorrow.
- "This path is quest within oneself." Thinking man questions:
  Who am I?
  Why am I here?
  Where do I belong?
  What is the purpose of my life?
  How am I responsible for my present state of being?
- This path is :
  - *Realistic* – Life is not a dream.
  - *Dualistic* – *Purusha* (Soul) and *Prakruti* (Nature) are two independent *elements.*
  - *Pluralistic* – No two Souls are the same.
- It guides an individual through Eternal Truth.
- It takes one's Soul to achievement of *bliss and enlightenment.*
- It brings stability and balance in life.
- It specifies that it is knowledge that leads to state of illumination.
- It leads towards self achievement through the process of self analysis and self realization.

"Gyan Yoga is path of Soul searching—The Way of Wisdom"

4. Mantra Yoga: Union by sound and voices

- A *"mantram"* is a sound (a mass of radiant energy) that has a particular effect on mind and body.
- *"Mann"* means mind, *"Tra"* means freedom. It frees the mind from desires.
- Mantra also means "self talk" which leads to fearlessness and improves self-esteem.
- The practice of Mantra Yoga influences consciousness through repeating (aloud and inwardly) certain syllables, words or phrases (mantras).
- **How the Mantra Yoga has evolved?**
  It is said that the relationship of a word to the object it (the word) denotes, is eternal, not arbitrary and there is a system of every "natural sound" for everything in the Universe.
- *Shastras* (Indian Philosophy) say that Mantras should be used only if one is a vegetarian. The body chemistry is completely different when a vegetarian diet is followed as is the effect of mantra practice.
- The repeated recitation of Mantras is *"Japa"*.
- I strongly believe in two Mantras: **SOHAM and AUM.**
  ### a. SOHAM:
  It is *Ajapa* Mantra: Unconscious Repetitive Prayer.
  SOHAM – *"Sah"* means 'He' and *"Aham"* means 'I'. The immortal spirit am I.
  Every living creature unconsciously breathes this prayer with each inward breath.
  HAMSAH – "I am He"; this is with each outgoing breath.
  Continuous recitation of SOHAM goes on forever with each living creature throughout his life.
  He offers every breath of his being to the Lord as a sacrifice and receives the breath of life from the Lord as his blessings.

This mantra signifies practice of Pranayama where *Pran*, vital force of individual energy, harmonizes with the cosmic energy.

This mantra has great therapeutic effects in prevention and cure of **respiratory, circulatory and nervous system** diseases.

b. AUM:

- It is **Mahamantra**, most highly regarded mantra.
- It resides in our forehead says our Shastras.
- It is composed of three sounds, comprising three states of consciousness.
- It is composed on three syllables, namely the letters AUM and when spoken, it has a crescent and a dot on the top.

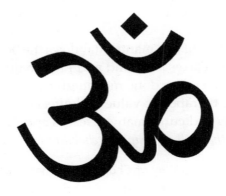

Fig. 5.5: The "Aum" mantra with crescent and dot on the top

'A'

- *Pronounced with open mouth.*
- Represents waking state.
- Symbolizes speech.
- Absence of desire.
- Past tense
- **G** —Lord Brahma: The Generator

'U'

- *Pronounced with partially closed mouth.*
- Represents dreamy state.
- Symbolizes the mind.
- Absence of fear.
- Present tense
- **O** - Lord Vishnu: The Operator

'M'

- *Pronounced with closed mouth.*
- Represents deep sleep.
- Symbolizes breath of life.
- Absence of anger.
- Future tense
- **D** - Lord Mahesh: The Destroyer

GOD – represents divinity – **AUM** prevails in whole universe.

- The recitation of this mantra <u>stabilizes</u> the body, <u>regulates</u> the breath, <u>relaxes</u> the mind and <u>illuminates</u> the soul.
- It's recitation when done meaningfully and properly has enormous therapeutic value and effects.
- It prevents and cures many diseases and disorders.
- *It leads to the path of complete rehabilitation.*

"Mantra Yoga – The Way of Chanting Rhymes, Songs, Recited words have great power to heal oneself and others"

5. Hath Yoga: Union by bodily mastery

- The word *Hatha is* derived from two roots:
  "*Ha*" means "*sun*", *positive male current*, located in the naval area.
  "*Tha*" means "moon", *negative female current*, located in the head region.
- The flow of breath in the right nostril is called '*sun breath*' and the flow of breath in left nostril is the '*moon breath.*'

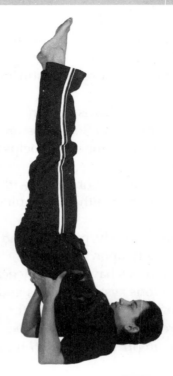

Fig. 5.6: Sarvangasana—The shoulder stand pose Hathyoga.
The way of physical mastery

- *Hatha* is thus harmonizing of the two energies of the body and regulating the breath, mind and body.
- It is also called as the Physiological **Yoga or Yoga of Vitality.**
- It is the later development of all forms of Yoga.
- It is not a path of physical discipline which is done forcefully or extensively as the name implies.
- *Saint Swatmaram* is the founder of this path who says that "Hathyoga is the attainment of perfect *Rajyoga.*" **It is the staircase of Rajyoga.**
- The ultimate goal of this path is "Kundalini Jagran" i.e. awakening the dormant potential energy located in the base of the spine.

- The means to reach this goal are through *Asana* (Postures), *Pranayama* (Breath Regulation) and *Mudras* (Body parts' positioning).
- It's best known feature is posturing – in particular sitting–
  - *Padmasana* – the Lotus Posture.
  - *Shirsana* – the Head Stand Posture.
- It is viewed as a hygiene which helps in purification of total organism.
- It is the most practical of Yogas with its emphasis on procuring Vibrant health and tapping the organism's latent energy.
- It works upon the body, purifying and perfecting it and through the body upon the mind.
- *Hathayoga* exercises have their practical benefits to the health of **nervous system, glands and vital organs.**
- Six impediments (obstructions) for pursuit of Hath Yoga are *excessive food, labour, speech, bathing with cold water, night eating, fasting, sociability and unsteadiness.*
- Six requirements for the pursuit of Hath Yoga are – *Enthusiasm, Courage, Patience, Knowledge, Determination and Solitude.*

"Whether young, old, or lean, one who discards laziness gets success if he practises Yoga. Practice alone is the means of success" – the way of Physical Mastery.

6. **Raj Yoga: Union by mental mastery**
   - It is believed to be the Royal (Raj) path, which is widely accepted and practised worldwide.
   - It is natural, simple, rational, practical, non-invasive and non-addictive path.
   - It's ultimate goal is Illumination (Samadhi) through *self-analysis and self-realization.*

- It is also called as *Yoga of Meditation.*
- It is closely associated with the systematization of Yoga techniques by Patanjali (second century B.C) by Bhagwan Patanjali.
- It works upon the mind, refining and perfecting it and through the mind upon the body.
- It is the easiest way to abolish negativity in life and make our mind think positively.
- It is the architect of *Inner Self.*
- Mastery over "Self" is Rajyoga.
- It proposes to put before humanity a practical and philosophical and scientifically approved method of reaching the Truth.
- It trains the mind and enables it to know its own nature.
- Its practice illuminates the *principles, values and attitudes* in life and inculcates morality in life.
- It helps to regulate the rhythm and rate of mind thereby our body with love and understanding.
- The mind is the "king of senses". One who has conquered the mind, senses, passions, thoughts and reason is a king amongst men. He is fit for RajYoga – the royal union with the universal spirit.
- This path of Yoga is the fountain for the other three paths of *Karma, Bhakti* and *Gyan.*
- It brings calmness and tranquility and prepares the mind for "Absolute Self surrender to God."
- Its goal can be reached through the eight limbs (stages) of Yoga of which the best-known features are the Meditative Asanas (Posturing).

"Raj Yoga is Thinking spiritually and Living peacefully – the way of Spiritual Practice."

CRISS CROSSING OF YOGA PATHS

Analyzing, interpreting and integrating the brief summary of some of the main Yoga systems mentioned above, one can perceive that it would be difficult to practise any one of them without to some extent incorporating features from others.

- Concentration: A central feature of Raj Yoga operates in all other paths in varying degrees.
- Devotion: A central feature of Bhakti Yoga provides effective feeling in all other paths.
- Selfless Service: A central feature of Karma Yoga, integrates devotion and knowledge to reach to the Supreme union.
- Knowledge: The central feature of Gyan Yoga leads to the destination of Absolute Truth.

"Truth prevails. There is no religion higher than truth."

6   THE ASHTANG YOGA

"He would not be the emperor of the world, who conquers the whole world or all nations, but he would be the slave of ambition. But he, who conquers his own mind, is the real conqueror of the world."

— Gautam Buddha

Those who practise Raj Yoga with its proper knowledge of science and theory as well as of Psychology and Philosophy, gain sound health and perfect mind along with the living inspiration of entering into the states of concentration (*Dharna*) and meditation (*Dhyana*).

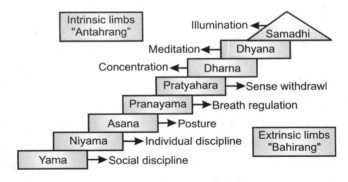

Fig. 6.1: Sage Patanjali's ashtang yoga ladder

THE STUDENTS OF YOGA

The students of Raj yoga can be divided into three classes:

1. **The Awakened Souls:**
   - They are born Yogis with pure souls.
   - Nothing in this world attracts their mind.
   - Nothing can obstruct their progress.
   - They just meditate regularly (Abhyas and Vairagya).

2. **The Half Awakened Souls:**
   - They need more experience.
   - They do not know exactly what they want, hence cannot make steady progress.
   - They find great many obstacles, as their mind is always disturbed.
   - In long run they can attain to highest goal through constant practise (Tapa, Swadhyaya, Ishwar Pranidhana).

3. **The Unawakened Souls:**
   - They have no spiritual ideals and live on animal plane.
   - The sense of desires and pleasures are highest ideals of their lives.
   - Their obstacles are stronger than their desires.
   - It is for these souls, the Ashtang Yoga Ladder is the means to reach the goal.
   - If they climb the steps faithfully, then wonderful results would come.

This science is the most practical of all the applied sciences and is the most beneficial to mankind under all conditions and circumstances.

This science can be practised by individuals of any religion, caste, color, and gender at any age to govern their daily actions of their earthly existence.

THE YOGA SUTRAS OF PATANJALI

The Yoga Sutra of Patanjali is divided into four chapters.

1. **Samadhi:**
   - Describes the nature of Yoga. It specifies on "the power of concentration."
   - Unless mind is stabilized the self will remain disturbed.
2. **Saadhan:**
   - Describes methods of regaining peace for "disturbed self."
   - The methods of relaxing "The Self " are Yama, Niyama, Asana, Pranayama, Pratyahara.
3. **Vibhuti:**
   - Enumerates the powers that a Yoga student comes across in his quest.
   - It is through the Dharna, Dhyana and Samadhi.
4. **Kevalya:**
   - Deals with state of enlightenment.

THE EIGHT LIMBS OF ASHTANG YOGA

The first five steps of the ladder are called as Bahiranga (Extrinsic) and the last three steos are called as Antahrang (Intrinsic)."

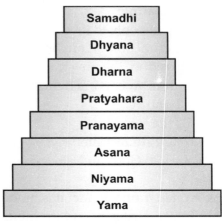

Fig. 6.2: Eight limbs and the psychosomatic approach

1. <u>YAMA: Social Discipline</u>

- These social norms if not obeyed bring chaos, violence and untruth.
- The roots of these evils are in greed, desire and attachment.
- They only bring pain and ignorance.
- Yama means restraints or moral disciplinary actions.
- The five such norms are:
  a. *Ahimsa*: **Non violence:**
     - Do not harm anyone in thought, speech and actions.
     - Violence is a state of mind and not of body or deed.
     - Violence arises from fear, weakness and ignorance.
     - One should be free of fear and anger.
     - Non-violence leads to nobility.
  b. *Satya:* **Truth:**
     - Be truthful to yourself and others.
     - It is the highest role of conduct or morality.
     - Truth in thought, speech and action.
     - Truth wins all battles.
     - Truth leads to politeness and firmness – A quality of healer.
  c. *Asteya:* **Non-Stealing:**
     - Non-stealing not only that belongs to others but also not to have attraction on anyone's belongings.
     - It teaches to reduce the physical needs to minimum.
     - It is freedom from craving, temptations.
     - It leads to honesty.
     - It tranquils the mind.
  d. *Brahmacharya:* **Life of Celebacy:**
     - Brahma means 'God' and Charya means 'focused upon'.
     - It is over rated Yama. In fact it is moderation in sex.
     - It is not forced austerity and prohibition.

- It is to follow divinity in thought, speech and action.
- With it, one develops a feeling of vitality and energy.

e. *Aparigraha:* **Non-acquisitiveness.**
  - Be indifferent and unattracted to materialistic things.
  - It is to be free from hoardings.
  - It aspires towards simplicity and faith in God.
  - It nurtures contentment.

"Yama are universal, moral commandments and followed everywhere."

2. <u>NIYAMA: Individual Discipline</u>

- The second limb of the Ashtang yoga ladder - The pillar: The Progress.
- They are rules of conduct towards oneself.
- They are to be followed positively and punctually.
- The five Niyamas are:

a. *Saucha:* **Cleanliness:**
  - Internal and external purification of mind and body.
  - Purification of body depends on fresh food, water and air.
  - Mental purity by friendliness, compassion, delight and disregard.
  - Cleanliness gives joy and radiance.
  - It leads to benevolence, peace, and unity with all.

b. *Santosh:* **Contentment:**
  - One who lives happily in congenial / non-congenial situations and atmosphere.
  - It is to be cultivated.
  - It leads to concentration and onepointedness.
  - Contentment and tranquility complement each other.

c. *Tapas:* **Penance – Austerity.**
  - Conquest of desires by thoughts, speech and action.

- It involves purification, self discipline and austerity.
- It builds character.
- Life without Tapas, is like heart without love.
- Tapas lead to wisdom, courage and simplicity.

d. *Swadhyaya:* **Self study:**
- "Swa" means 'self' and "adhyaya" means 'education'.
- It is education of life through self study.
- There is no sermonizing; one heart speaks to other.
- It tranquilises the mind, relaxes the body and nourishes the soul.
- It puts an end to ignorance and brings knowledge.

5. *Ishwar Pranidhana:* **Surrender to God:**
- Surrendering one's total self for all actions and will.
- It leads to acceptance of all situations. It is surrendering "I and mine" and passion.
- It leads to mental power and illumination.
- It reflects divinity within oneself.

"Niyamas performed with sincerity and dedication tranquilise, cheer and control the mind."

3. ASANAS: Postures and Positions

- The third limb: "the psychosomatic lubricating machine."
- *Asana* is a state of being and not doing.
- *Asana* is a state of stable body where mind also remains relaxed, happy and light.
- *Asana* conserves energy as it is an effortless act.
- *Asana* is a state where mind and body complement each other.
- *Asana* is a temple for the soul to reside.

"Asanas are for developing one's spiritual being and not just for fitness and disease cure."

"True Asana is that in which the thought of Brahma (God) flows effortlessly through the mind of Sadhak—The Yoga Student."

History of Yoga Asana

The names of Asana are significant and illustrate the principle of evolution. They have evolved over the centuries so as to exercise every muscle, nerve and gland in the body. These are being practised since more than 4000 years and are thousands in number of which 36 postures – Asanas are practised everywhere.

Rishis have invented them from *nature and surrounding*. The name of the Asana is significant and illustrates the *principle of evolution*. They are so named as, these on which and whom they were named never had illness or disease. Some are named after:

a. *Vegetation:* Vrikshasana (tree pose), Padmasana (lotus posture)
b. *Insects*: Salabhasana (locust pose), Vrischikasana (scorpion)
c. *Birds*: Kukutasana (cock), Mayurasana (peacock)
d. *Animals*: Ushtarsana (camel), Simhasana (lion)
e. *Aquatic animals*: Matsyasana (fish), Mandukasana (frog)
f. *Serpents*: Bhujangasana (cobra), Sarpasana (snake)
g. *Legendary heroes*: Virbhadrasana, Hanumanasana
h. *Sages*: Bharadvajasana, Kapilasana
i. *Mechanics*: Setubandhasana (bridge), Chakrasana (wheel)
j. *Body mechanics*: Janushirasana (head to knee), Uttanpadasana (bilateral SLR)

Classification of Asana

As per the progress, advancement and research on these asanas they are broadly classified based on –
a. Objectives – Meditation, Relaxation, Health.
b. Position of body – Sitting, Standing, Lying.

c. Body segment position.

d. Complimentory postures.

a. Objectives of Asanas:

i. *Meditative Postures: Spiritual Health*

Padmasana – for purity and holiness (Fig. 6.3A).

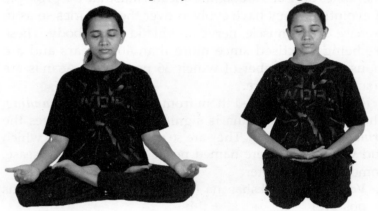

(A) Padmasana   **(B)** Vajrasana (The thunderbolt posture)

Fig. 6.3: Meditative asanas

Vajrasana – for firmness of mind and body (Fig. 6.3B).
Swastikasana – for noble thoughts, deeds and action.
Sukhasana - for tranquility and comfort.

- These are all sitting postures, where spine is in erect position maintaining its all curves.
- The body is in perfect, stable, steady posture.
- *Withdrawing attention from all materialistic desires.*
- Mind concentration within – with onepointedness – Ekagrata.
- Breath and mind regulation and control.
- Maximum benefit for "Spiritual upliftment" as mind is able to contemplate with Infinity.
- Improves physical, mental and social health of an individual.

"Self transformation leads to transformation of any situation"

ii. *Relaxation Postures: Mental health (Fig. 6.5)*

Shavasana: For progressive muscular relaxation (corpse posture) (Fig. 6.4)

Makarasana: Relaxation through energy conservation (crocodile posture).

Balkasana: Relaxed mind leads to relaxed body (infant posture) (Fig. 6.5).

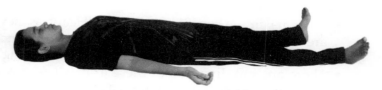

Fig. 6.4: Relaxation asana—Shavasana

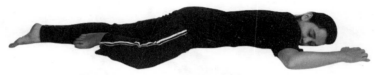

Fig. 6.5: Relaxation asana—Balkasana—The child posture

- These are all lying postures where relaxation of key points (proximal) of control leads to distal relaxation.
- These asana should be performed in between other asanas.
- One should not fall asleep while one is in this asana.
- Eyes should be closed though children may keep them open.
- These asanas have maximum effect on *mental relaxation*, through mind body concept as regulation of thoughts regulates the body, thereby improving stress coping mechanism.
- These asanas are also called as *"Stress Inoculators"* hence best for all *Psychomatic disorders*.
- They make the person more fresh and energetic.
- They improve physical as well as social health too.

iii. *Cultural postures: Physical health (Fig. 6.6):*

- These Asanas are performed in sitting, standing and lying positions (fundamental starting positions and derived postures).
- This group include maximum number of asanas.
- These asanas culture the individual physically in order to prepare the basis for Pranayama, Dhyana, etc.
- Their maximum benefit is on Physical Health as they are meant for reconditioning of the body and mind so as to bring stability, peace and sense of well being.
- There are sub-divisions of these asanas based on position of body and working pattern.

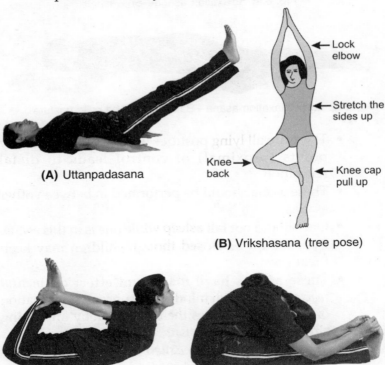

(A) Uttanpadasana

Lock elbow

Stretch the sides up

Knee back

Knee cap pull up

(B) Vrikshasana (tree pose)

(C) Dhanurasana (bow pose)   (D) Paschimottanasana (back stretch)

Fig. 6.6: Cultural asanas

b. Position of the Body (Fig. 6.7):

Table 6.1: Asanas—Classification as per body position

Lying		Sitting	Standing
Supine	Prone		
Uttanpadasana	Salbhasana	Parvatasana	Tadasana-fundamental standing posture
Pawanmuktasana	Dhanurasana	Gaumukhasana	Uttanasana
Setubandhasana	Bhujangasana	Veerasana	Uttkatasana
Shavasana	Makarasana	Padmasana	Vrikshasana
		All Meditative	Utthitasana
	Sarpasana	Shashankasana	Bharajdvasana
		Yogmudrasana	Upasthanasana
		Janu shirasana	Padhastasana

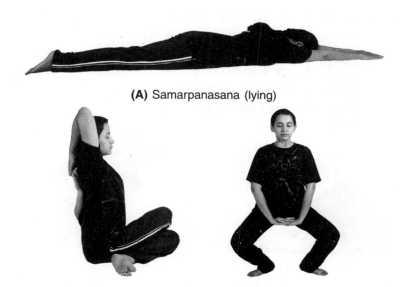

(A) Samarpanasana (lying)

(B) Gaumukhasana (sitting)   **(C)** Uthitasana (standing)

Fig. 6.7: Classification of asana—Body positions

c. Body Segment Position (Fig. 6.8):

Table 6.2: Asanas—Body segment position

Bending	Twisting	Topsyturvy
Forward Bending: Padhastasana	Vakrasana	Sarvangasana
Backward Bending: Upasthanasana	Ardhamatsyendrasana	Shirsasana
Side Bending: Trikonasana	Yogmudrasana I and II	Halasana

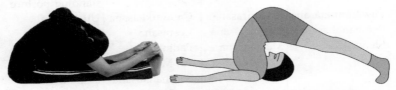

(A) Paschimotanasana (Bending)   **(B)** Modified Halasana (Topsy turvy)

Fig. 6.8: Classification of asana—Body segments positions

d. Complimentory Postures (Fig. 6.9):

- These Asanas compliment each other focusing on a fixed segment of Spinal column.
- E.g. Segment: Lumbo sacral joints of spine
  Backward Bend: Ushtrasana (camel pose) (Fig. 6.9A)
  Forward Bend: Paschhimottanasana (back stretch) (Fig. 6.9B)

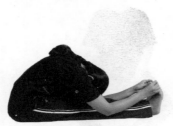
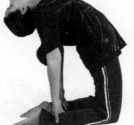

(A) Forward bend   **(B)** Backward bend

Fig. 6.9: Complimentary asanas

"Their objective is to regulate and balance by co-contraction and reciprocal relaxation of the muscles. These postures mobilize the spinal joints in both its directions, improving mobility too."

BENEFITS OF ASANAS

1. *Physical:*
   a. *Meditative asanas* help in regulating all the biological processes of body like blood pressure, heart rate, respiratory rate, digestion, metabolism, endocrine functions, etc.
   b. *Relaxation asanas* help in developing a state of homeostatis: physiological balance between the endocrine and autonomic nervous system.
   c. *Cultural asanas* recondition various joints, muscles, tendons, ligaments as well as reflex mechanism in order to offer a stable and comfortable posture for higher practise.

2. *Mental:*
   a. *Meditative asanas* decrease Rajas (Hyperactivity) and Tamas (inertia) gunas and increase Sattva Guna (purity) thereby tranquilizing the mind for higher achievements.
   b. *Relaxation asanas* render the mind more balanced and steady and aims at releasing tension working at the level of consciousness.
   c. *Cultural asanas* bring about an equilibrium in overall functioning including ego, emotions, behaviour and perception.

3. *Health:*
   a. *Meditative asanas* control or reduce all psychological disorders like migraine, headache, blood pressure problems, coronary artery diseases, gastric problems, ulcerative colitis, low back aches, rheumatism, etc.
   b. *Relaxation asanas* overcome mental as well as physical fatigue preventing all overuse syndromes or repetitive trauma syndromes.
   c. *Cultural asanas* main objective is on body functions, thereby improving overall functions of musculo-

skeletal, respiratory, neuromuscular, gynaecological and skin conditions.

4. *Spiritual:*
   a. *Meditative asanas* help in illuminating the hidden potential vital source of energy – Prana.
   b. *Relaxation asanas* help in developing "feeling of surrender" thereby always give a feeling of joy and bliss.
   c. *Cultural asanas'* main objective is psychophysical. It directs the mind within and works on eternal principle of energy conservation for higher upliftment of body mind and soul.

PRE-REQUISITES FOR ASANAS

(i). *Necessities for doing Yogasanas:*
   a. *Self Inclination:* One should have interest for one's own development. It should not be practised forcefully.
   b. *Guidance under* Yoga teacher: One should do with proper assessment and under guidance. Practising asanas by watching television and reading books directly are not appropriate which would otherwise invite unwanted problems. No two individuals are same.
   c. *Regularity:* One should practise asana with regularity, sincerity and psycho physically. Continuity should be maintained throughout life for long lasting results.
   d. *Concentration:* Without concentration nothing can be achieved. Concentration leads to self determination and confidence.
(ii). *Mind involvement:*
   a. Mind should be *peaceful* and *happy*.
   b. Yogic warm up for *preparedness* before asana is an important aspect.
   c. While performing the asana, *think* *of its benefit* simultaneously.

d. *Quality of being* in an asana is important rather than the long period of unstable, exhaustive holding of asana.

e. *Feeling of lightness* experience is must rather than exhaustion after the release of asana.

(iii). *Some practisal tips for Yogasanas:*

a. *Atmosphere:* should be silent and peaceful.

b. *Cleanliness:* bladder should be empty; bowel must be evacuated for better results. Bath should be taken before practising and bath after practising aids in relaxation of the mind and body.

c. *Food:* vegetarian diet for higher achievements. Empty stomach is a must approximately with one, to one and a half hours after snacks, four hours after meals. Food may be taken half – an – hour after asana.

d. *Water:* in between, before and after it can be as per requirement.

e. *Place:* should be ventilated, clean and quiet. It should not be performed on bare floor or uneven surface but on a folded blanket or mattress.

f. *Time:* the best suitable time is early morning or late evening. In morning the mind is fresh but the body is stiff so regular practise in morning improves work efficiency and mental determination powers. In the evening the mind is exhausted but body is flexible so regular practise in the evening replenishes the mind and body with energy, removing fatigue and making one feel fresh, at ease and calm.

g. *Position:* the position should be preferably facing the East or the North.

h. *Age:* it can be practised by all age groups but children less than 12 years old age should not practise vigorously the Cultural asana as the body organs are under formation age.

i. *Clothing:* should be clean, simple, and suitable to the climate and of loose fitting. It should not obstruct or restrict any body positions.

j. *Rest:* Occasional short periods of rest between the practise period leads to long lasting effects as it avoids fatigue syndromes.

k. *Breath:* Regulation of breath should be through nostrils and as per the required anatomical body position, conserves energy to produce significant results.

l. *Caution:* no undue stress or strain should fall on face muscles, eyes, ears and breathing patterns.

m. *Precaution:*
   • Beginner should perform with eyes open to know and correct the errors.
   • Later on eyes can be shut as one gains control.
   • Women: No balancing postures should be performed on hands. During pregnancy all asanas should be practised under supervision.
   • Illness: Asana should not be taken up abruptly after a prolonged illness.
   • Do not control urine or stool during practise.
   • Remember all contraindications of each asana.
   • Physical exercises like swimming, aerobics, walking should not be followed immediately before or after asana.

"Asana nourish and strengthen self confidence and give a feeling of well being, hence regularity, continuity and patience in their practise are very necessary."

4. PRANAYAMA: The Yogic Breathing

• It is the fourth limb of Asthang yoga ladder. Pranayama is also "silencing the breath". It is also called as the Soul of Yoga Science.

- Prana is vital source of energy, it is the motivating element of earth and is source of origin of a thought. "Prana" also means "breath, respiration, life, vitality, wind or strength".

"Ayama" means to regulate, to restrain, to control, to channelise and to stretch."

Pranayama is to inspire, motivate, regulate and balance the vital force that is in the body for a long, healthy and happy life.

Hath Yoga describes about eight varieties of Pranayama and its objective for Pranayama is for physical results and Kundilini Jagran (The spiritual awakening). ˙

Raj Yoga records only four types of Pranayama, the distinction being based on the nature of retention of breath (Kumbhaka) and its objective is psychical results.

This control is upon all the functions of breathing namely:

1. Inhalation: Puraka: Filling up the lungs.
2. Retention: Antara-Kumbhaka: Holding the breath within.
3. Exhalation: Rechaka: Emptying the lungs.
4. Retention: Bahiya-Kumbhaka: Holding the breath without.

- *A Yogi's life is not measured by the number of his days but by the number of his breaths.*
- A slow rhythmic deep breathing leads to longetivity of life..
- Yoga believes that perfect control over the mind and the body can be reached by controlling the motions of the lungs. The center which regulates the respiration is the controlling power over the other centers. Pranayama not only controls the breath but also is the vital force in the most scientific method and pattern.

PRE-REQUISITES OR PRACTICAL TIPS FOR PRANAYAMA

- It should be practised under guidance and supervision.
- It should be practised in clean airy space.
- It should be practised in complete solitude and in a quiet place.
- Best time is early morning, before sunrise but can be practised in evening too after sunset.
- Period of practise should be about 15 minutes a day for common man and as per one's capacity. Mastery of Pranayama is 80 cycles per session.
- Best position is sitting on floor on a blanket or mattress.
- Best asana for practising is Padmasana (lotus pose)
- Better practised with empty stomach. Milk can be taken 15-20 minutes before the session but to be practised only after six hours of meals. After completion of Pranayama, light food can be taken after an hour.
- Do not bathe immediately after practise.
- It should be practised always before asanas with a considerable time in between them.
- If one is exhausted in between, then the cycles should not be practised continuously.

"Regulated rhythmic breathing is an important pre-requisite for Pranayama:"

Beginning with inhalation: exhalation	1:1
Progression	1:2
Progression – inhalation: retention:exhalation	1:1:2
Gradual Progression –	1:2:2
Mastery – inhalation:retention:exhalation	1:4:2

- Pranayama is always begun for the first time in spring or autumn.
- It should be practised through nose and should not cause strain on any muscle.

- Eyes should always be closed for concentration within.
- Knowledge of all three Bandhs (locks) is necessary for its practise:

Jalandhar Bandh – Chin lock – after inhalation.

Uddiyan Bandh – Abdominal lock – during exhalation.

Mool Bandh – Perenial lock – all three phases.

Classification of Pranayama

a. Patanjali's Yoga Sutra: Based on Kumbhaka
1. *Bahyakumbhaka:* Retention after Exhalation.
2. *Antarkumbhaka:* Retention after Inhalation.
3. *Sthambhvritti:* Retention during any phase of Inhalation or Exhalation.
4. *Kevalkumbhaka:* Ultimate mastery of Retention in any phase.

b. Hathyoga Pradipika: Eight Varieties
1. *Suryabhedana:* Energize the mind and body.
2. *Ujjayi:* Royal breathing for triumph and victory.
3. *Sitkari:* Has cooling effect on body.
4. *Shitali:* Cools the systems, soothes the eyes and ears.
5. *Bhastrika:* Bellow breaths for digestive functions and cleansing effect.
6. *Bhramari:* Large bee humming for insomnia relief.
7. *Moorchha:* Facilitates senses withdrawal.
8. *Plavani:* The floating breath.

Suryabhedan and Ujjayi *should be practised in winter only.* Shitali and Sitkari *in summer.* Bhastrika *round the year.*

c. Pronounciation
1. Sagarbha: with enchanting mantra or rhymes. Example: Aum, Soham.
2. Agarbha: without mantras one should practise regularly with the above mentioned rhythm.

d. The Cleansing Pranayama
Anulom vilom : It is also known as "Nadi shodhan Pranayama".

Benefits of Pranayama

• Amount of oxygen consumed during Pranayama is less than the oxygen consumed in normal breathing. Therefore it is wrong to say that Pranayama requires more oxygen.

• It neither produces any emotion nor it expresses any thought or desire, hence its main function or advantage is Energy conservation. Normally most of the energy of an individual is wasted in baseless thoughts and uncontrolled desires.

• One becomes more connected to reality with its regular practise; hence it is a prime mean of rehabilitation.

• "Living in reality and accepting the circumstances with positivity, in spite of disability is REHABILITATION."

1. *Physical:*
   a. Cleanses all tubular channels of the body.
   b. One gets habituated to deep breathing technique, hence a good gas exchange, which leads to good transportation of oxygenated blood to all tissues of body. Always a feeling of freshness and vitality.
   c. Has significant benefit on Cardiovascular system also, as reserve capacity of lungs is increased.
   d. Digestive function also improves. Facilitate absorption function of small intestine and large intestine.
   e. Liver and Kidney functions also strengthen as they are dependent on maximum supply of oxygenated blood.
   f. Reconditioning of Neural tissues, Respiratory center in brain gets stimulated; thereby Autonomic nervous system activity is balanced and improves.

    g. Regulation of the internal environment (systems) of the body.

2. *Mental:*
   a. Slow, rhythmic, regulated breathing regulates and controls the thoughts process and eventually the mind.
   b. Breath is the connecting link between the mind and the body.
   c. Mind relaxes and experiences a feeling of serenity.
   d. Concentration level improves.
   e. Unveils the curtain of ignorance, hence outlook improves.
   f. Memory, learning, perception ability also improve.
   g. Will power and determination strengthens.

3. *Social:*
   a. Interpersonal relationship improves as one's perception and acceptance improves.
   b. Adjustment and accommodativeness with everyone and all situations.
   c. Nourishes a feeling of "To Bear", "To Care" and "To Share".
   d. Encourages one "To live and let live".
   e. Atmosphere in the family, community and society becomes conducive, hence communication become more transparent and easy.
   f. Harmonizing the mind with body cultivates harmony everywhere.

4. *Spiritual:*

   "Asana eradicate diseases of the body, and Pranayama eradicates sins of the mind".

   a. One gets rid of the vices of lust, passion, greed, possessiveness anger, arrogance, etc.

b. One is blessed with sattva guna-Harmony.

c. It leads to Spiritual awakening.

d. Inner voice begins to be heard.

e. Concept of "Self" develops leading to self realization.

f. A state of "Poise and bliss" in all situations.

"Pranayama can be considered as most powerful weapon to combat any disease and win the battle for rehabilitation."

Types of Pranayama

The classification has been discussed. Here in this text two types of Pranayama are discussed which can be practised by any person of any age, sex, disease, discomfort without any limitations and contraindications.

i. *Anulom-Vilom Pranayama: The Alternate nostril breathing.*

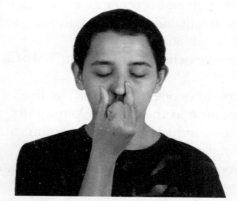

Fig. 6.10: Pranayama: Anulom Vilom—Hand position

Introduction:

• It is one of the eight types of Pranayama as per Hathyogpradipika.

• It can be practised with "kumbhaka" or "without kumbhaka".

- It is also known as "Nadi shodhan" when practised without kumbhaka, as it has cleansing effect on all the channels of the body.
- It is also known as the "Sun and Moon breath"

The Rationale:

- The Sun (positive energy) and Moon (negative energy) *are equalized and harmonized.*
- The sympathetic and parasympathetic effects *on the air channels are balanced hence there is regulated rhythmic breathing as air flow is free and fair.*
- The two energy current effects of heating (pingala) and cooling (ida) *are neutrilised, giving the effect of channel purification.*

Technique

- **Posture:** • Any comfortable meditative posture, preferably Padmasana.
  - Spine straight but relaxed.
  - Abdomen slightly tucked in.
  - Hand position: left on the left knee and right thumb to close right nostril. And right little and ring finger to close left nostril.
- **Eyes:** Closed
- **Mind:** On **Anahat chakra**—The chest region
- **Breath:** • Close the right nostril.
  - Empty the lungs by exhaling through the left nostril.
  - Inhale through left nostril.
  - Close the left nostril.
  - Exhale through the right nostril.
  - Inhale through the right nostril.
  - Close the right nostril.
  - Exhale through the left nostril.

This completes one cycle of alternate nostril breathing.

- Such cycles can be practised gradually as per the capacity of a person.
- Maintain the rest of the principles of Pranayama as explained earlier.
- The practise should be initially done under supervision.

"Anulom vilom Pranayama when practised with retention, then wisely use of Bandhs should be advocated."

- **Rest:** After practise rest in shavasana for some time.
  Advantages
  1. Cleansing effect on all channels of energy within body.
  2. Relaxing effect on mind and body.
  3. Regulates all vital signs of the body, i.e. Blood pressure, Heart rate, Respiratory rate and Temperature.
  4. Therapeutic effects on
     - Neuromuscular disorder like parkinsonian syndrome.
     - Cardiovascular disorder like Coronary artery disease
     - Respiratory disorder like Bronchial Asthma.
     - Musculoskeletal disorder like Painful syndromes.
     - All issues of women and during pregnancy too.
     - All other psychosomatic disorders.

"This breathing technique has a role in esoteric Yoga connected with the arousal and control of latent psychic force and fluctuations"

— Shiv Samhita

ii. *Ujjayi Pranayama: The victorious breathing:*
    Introduction:
    - It is also one of the eight types of Pranayama as explained in Hathyogpradipika.
    - "Utt" means "to elevate" and "Jay" means "victory".

- It elevates and uplifts oneself from the worldly desires and achieves victory over thought processes, the chitta
- It can be practised in all positions, during activities and, any time hence most practical of all the Pranayamas.

Special Features:

- Some texts suggest Inhalation through both the nostrils and exhalation through the left, having closed the right nostril.
- But mostly it is practised as inhalation through both and exhalation also through both the nostrils.
- The epiglottis (upjihva) is partly closed during inhalation and exhalation producing an audible sound.
- This is an "easy method of doing deep breathing".
- The abdomen is kept slightly contracted.

Technique:

- Posture: Any comfortable posture with spine and head erect, with hands cupped on the lap, or in Gyana mudra (pose) on both the knees.
- Preparatory phase: Exhale slowly through both the nostrils.
- One cycle: Inhale rhythmically and slowly through both the nostrils.

    Maintain perineal lock or moolbandh.

    The partially closed glottis allows the air to enter slowly with a soft audible sound.

    Hold with "the chin lock" till comfort level.

    Exhale slowly maintaining the abdominal lock, through both nostrils.

    Follow all the other recommendations of Pranayama practise.

The Ujjayi Shvasana (breathing):

- In any comfortable position of sitting lying or even standing.

- Continue the pattern of inhalation and exhalation without retention and locks.
- Concentrate on **Vishudhha** chakra—The throat region.
- Practised on the occasions of working, walking reading writing, etc.
- The most economical practical and beneficial breathing technique in day-to-day life.
- Great value in the therapeutic effect of cardiac patient's rehabilitation.

Advantages:

- Cleansing effect on the air channels of the respiratory passage.
- Reduces air flow resistance and turbulence.
- Improves thoracic mobility and chest expansion in all directions.
- Increases vital capacity.
- Richly oxygenates the blood.
- Removes phlegm.
- Tones the nervous system.
- Improves digestion.
- Therapeutic effect on Cardiovascular disorders specially in CABG Rehabilitation, Asthma prevention and cure, Neuralgias and Stroke Rehabilitation as no hand postures, in all Women issues mainly during Menorrhogia and Menopause and Geriatric Rehabilitation.

"Let the man perform Ujjayi to destroy decay and death."

— Gheranda Samhita

The main feature of any Pranayama is stilling of mind. It is it's over riding purpose.

"Pranayama is itself a form of meditation".

5. <u>PRATYAHAAR: Sense Withdrawal</u>

- It is to divert one's attention within by controlling the thought processes and desires.
- It is to be focused within – self analysis to self realization.
- It is connecting link between the Extrinsic limbs (Bahirang) – Yama, Niyama, Asana, Pranayama and the Intrinsic limbs (Antahrang) – Dharna, Dhyana and Samadhi. The connecting link between body and mind.
- "Easy to understand but very difficult to practise."

6. <u>DHARANA: Concentration</u>

"Only good in life is Concentration and only evil is Dissipation."

- Concentration is ability of an individual to fix up the mind to an idea, thought, or object.
- Concentration is diverting all energies on one focal point.
- Concentration or Dharna is sixth step or limb of the Ashtangyoga ladder. When the body is toned up by the asanas, mind is replenished by Pranayama, and the senses brought under control by pratyahara, the sadhaka , student of yoga, reaches this step of Dharna. Example of Arjuna provides us with an ideal meaning of what concentration is, in archery contest. He could only see the bird's eye, which was the target chosen by his Guru Drona.
  A. *Tratak: An easy method of concentration:*
    - It is one of the cleansing process of Shatkarmas, the six cleansing disciplines.
    - It is the simplest process for development of concentration.

- It consists of fixation of the eye with a stare without a blink on some object in front of the eye level. The object could be a small distinct point, deity or flame of candle, tip of the nose, toes or center of eyebrows. This fixation is till eye starts watering.
- Position: Any comfortable sitting position.
- Place: A quiet distraction free place.
- Time: Any time of the day but preferably morning.
- Duration: As per the ability and capacity of person approximately 15 to 20 minutes in a session.

Modification: For practising Tratak

- One can gaze steadily on an external object, but if there is too much eye watering, then try gazing within; visualize about the object to be concentrated upon. It takes some time, but eventually develops power over mental faculties. Initially the session may be short, but as one practises regularly the session may be lengthened.
- AUM or SOHAM mantra can be used as means for developing concentration power.

Advantages of Dharana:
- It is one of the best means to switch off sensory information.
- It helps in opening up of dormant centers in the brain.
- It is an easiest method in gradually setting up control over central nerves with its physiological and psychological considerations.
- It improves eyesight and other higher faculty functions of memory, decision making, reasoning, judgement, etc.
- Power of command develops. One is in control of one's own thought, speech and action.

- Harmony between mind and body develops.
- A state of Ekagrata, i.e. one pointedness develops.
- It strengthens the journey towards internal quest.

7. <u>DHYANA</u>: Meditation

"The greatest help to Spiritual life is Meditation. In meditation we divest ourselves of all material conditions and feel our divine nature. We do not depend upon any external help in meditation."

— Swami Vivekananda.

- Meditation is mastery over Attention.
- It is the seventh step of the Ashtangyoga ladder.
- This step can only be climbed by sincere and honest practise of the first six steps of the ladder.
- It is a state of emotional stability and quietening of mind-the primary requirement.

"When the flow of concentration is un interrupted, the state that arises is Meditation."

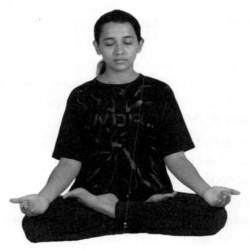

Fig. 6.11: Padmasana—The meditation pose

- Focus on self for long without disturbance of place, time and person.
- *Meditation* has features in common with muscular relaxation, autogenic training and biofeedback, but it is essentially different because all types of meditation operate distinctively through mental rather than physical modality.

Method and Prerequisites

- There have been many methods and techniques explained.
- Perfection in meditation cannot be gained by any mechanical means.
- *Meditation* is more of an experience than a scientific explanation.
- *It is not a recitation of sacred mantras.* These mantras are means to reach the state.
- A *quiet atmosphere* for the beginners. But the purpose of meditation is to be free absolutely of the external clutches of time, place, purpose, posture and even breathing.
- A comfortable sitting posture essentially with *spine erect*, and a meditative posture preferred with *face towards East or North.*

Time: *Sunrise, noon, sunset and midnight. At least two of these four should be utilized daily. It is observed by Yogis in India that during these four phases everything in nature enters spontaneously towards peace and tranquility.*

Attitude; Initially passive, just let things, events happen, let thoughts come and go, do not resist, just acknowledge. Do not force on concentration method.

Breathing: Gentle, smooth, slow, soundless, even, deep rhythmic and regulated. This tranquilises the mind and harmonizes the *SELF.*

"This practise begins at the physiological level with proper control of reflexes, postures and respiratory functions, progressing to techniques of concentration, and to the progressive control of the higher mental processes leading to a state of bliss."

Advantages of Dhyana

1. *It gives tranquility of mind,* thereby helps in tackling all types of problems with patience.
2. *A feeling of "Self worth" develops.* Behavioural patterns of hyperactivity, aggression, and rage decrease and creativity, enthusiasm and energy levels increase.
3. Quality of life improves.
4. Interpersonal and intrapersonal relationships strengthen.
5. *A feeling of "I am OK, you are OK and everything is OK"* develops which bring peace, prosperity and harmony.
6. A calm relaxed mind conserves energy, *developing positive health and harmony..*

These qualitative benefits definitely give quantitative effects on all the systems of the body, the results of which speak for itself without any experiments and proofs.

"Meditation leads to powerful heart, supple spine, strong and soft abdomen, sensual control and a state of bliss which is different from happiness or pleasure".

8. SAMADHI: Illumination

"A state of all consciousness, a highest individual state, a state with vibrant powers to motivate high intellect, will power, power of knowledge love, etc."

- It is the final stage, a superconscious state, *a state of self realization and actualization.*
- It is a *divine communion* state where the individual soul is united with the universal spirit and realizes the perfect oneness.

- It is the end of sadhaka's quest.
- It is a state of peak of meditation where *the body and senses are at rest, but the mind is alert.*
- *There is no sense of "I or mine".*
- *The mind is thoughtless and tongue is speechless.*
- *There is silence, "A Golden Silence".*

Obstacles to reach this state:

1. *Disease:* Body conscious person falls more sick.
2. *Laziness:* Person has low energy levels.
3. *Doubt:* Lack of faith in anything.
4. *Cessation of struggle:* Loss of interest.
5. *Desires:* Thirst for worldly pleasures.
6. *Heaviness:* Tiredness of body and mind.
7. *False knowledge:* Due to ignorance.
8. *Non-attainment of concentration:* Due to disease, laziness doubt.
9. *Falling away from attained state:* Due to lack of concentration, grief, sorrow, fear, physical causes like tremors, shivering, restlessness, irregular breathing also are obstacles.

Means of removing these obstacles:

- Meditation.
- Pranayama.
- Pratyahara.
- Regular practise of these with determination, dedication and devotion.

"Samadhi is self realization. ONENESS OF INTERNAL AND EXTERNAL WORLD. The Meditator, Act of meditation and Object meditated upon, all merge in one single vision. This leads to supreme happiness, free from complementary feelings".

Chapter 7

SHATCHAKRA—THE YOGIC WHEELS OF CONSCIOUSNESS

CHAKRA is a sanskrit word meaning *"WHEEL"*. These are spinning circles of energy and regions of mind power.

- The *shatchakra* or *"seven chakras"* or *"seven wheels of consciousness"* according to Yogic concepts are *psychophsiological centres* which work as staircase *to channelise the human potential energy (kundalini shakti) to progress upwards through each step of chakra for liberation.*

- Chakra and Nadi (energy channels) knowledge have surfaced in every society that followed, and nurtured the mystical tradition. It is quoted in Chinese Acupuncture system, American literature, Buddhists, Sikhs, Sufis and Christian sects, though named and explained in different aspects.

CHAKRAS CONNECTED WITH THE ACTIVITY OF PRANA WHICH FLOWS THROUGH THE NADIS

- These chakras are also called as wheels of consciousness of human potential energy.

- These chakras are *amplifiers and regulators of the vital force of energy of our body-THE PRANA.*

- These chakras as explained by the Yogis define……..
    - *our state of mind*
    - *our view and attitude in life*

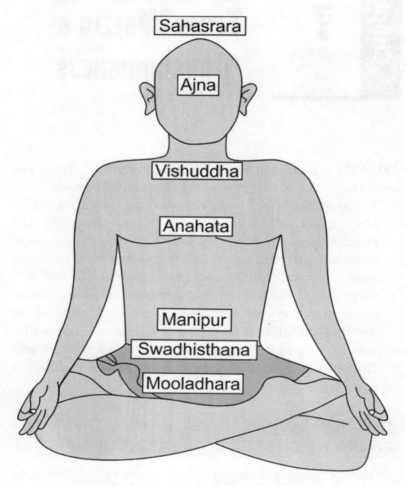

Fig. 7.1: The seven chakras—Body location

Each Higher Chakra Controls that Below it. This is the Law

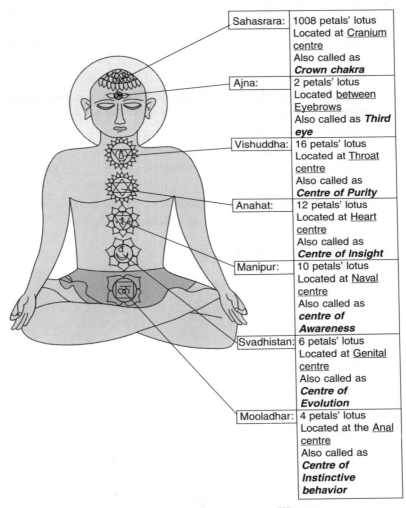

Sahasrara:	1008 petals' lotus Located at <u>Cranium centre</u> Also called as ***Crown chakra***
Ajna:	2 petals' lotus Located <u>between Eyebrows</u> Also called as ***Third eye***
Vishuddha:	16 petals' lotus Located at <u>Throat centre</u> Also called as ***Centre of Purity***
Anahat:	12 petals' lotus Located at <u>Heart centre</u> Also called as ***Centre of Insight***
Manipur:	10 petals' lotus Located at <u>Naval centre</u> Also called as ***centre of Awareness***
Svadhistan:	6 petals' lotus Located at <u>Genital centre</u> Also called as ***Centre of Evolution***
Mooladhar:	4 petals' lotus Located at the <u>Anal centre</u> Also called as ***Centre of Instinctive behavior***

Fig. 7.2: The Chakras—Energy Wheels' Functions

KUNDALINI JAAGRAN: THE AWAKENING...

- These chakras are part of *subtle body*.
- *The human potential energy when transforms to kinetic energy, and as it passes through all these chakras, while transcending upwards, the power and effect both are amazing, our ancient literature quotes.* The latent energy that is located at the base of spine, when channelised through these chakras, **leads the PRANA—*the vital force of energy towards bliss, happiness and liberation which the Yogic texts call as "kundilini jaagran" or "awakening".***
- According to *yoga*, this potential energy can be converted into kinetic form either *spontaneously* or by *meditation processes*. This transformation of human potential energy to kinetic energy is awakening. *Chakras are like transformers that regulate the flow of energy.*

Energy Currents of the Body

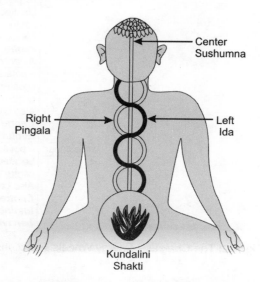

Fig. 7.3: Nadis—Energy currents of body

Energy is neither created nor destroyed, but is transformed from one state to another. **Chakras** serve the means of transformation of energy as per the requirement and necessity of human mind and body. If this energy is not transformed as per the requirement due to imbalance between the glandular functions and nervous plexuses, then it leads to improper functioning of body organs and systems, lowering the immune response. *The three main energy currents according to yogic science are...*

1. **Sushumna:**
   - It flows in the centre of the spinal cord (spinal canal CSF).
   - It is *spiritual in nature,* and flow directly through the spine and into the head.

2. **Ida:**
   - It flows to the *left of the spine.*
   - It is said to be the *feminine current.*
   - It is a *passive physical current.*
   - It is *materialistic in nature.*

3. **Pingala:**
   - It flows to the *right of the spine.*
   - It is said to be the *masculine current.*
   - It is *aggressive intellectual current.*
   - It is *mental in nature.*

Depending on the attitude and nature of each individual, the energy generally expresses itself as spiritual, physical or mental.

"Developing, energizing and strengthening the flow of Sushumna helps in prevention and elimination of all psychosomatic disorders and achieving PERFECT HEALTH".

CHAKRAS: THE PSYCHO-PHYSIOLOGICAL CENTRES

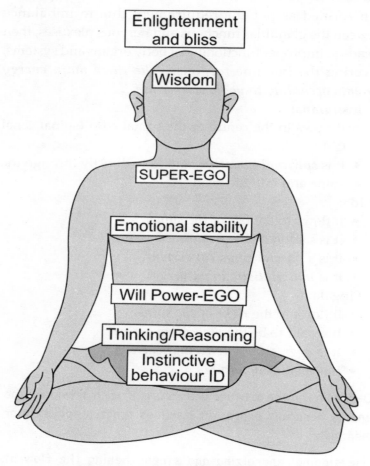

Fig. 7.4: Chakras—The Psychophysiological centre

- The personality complex contains *seven traits* that help in an individual's *education and development*.

- The self healing movement and therapies are nowadays focusing on the chakras as most of the idiopathic, chronic, non traumatic illnesses are Psychosomatic. The most modern medical practitioners also have started believing that senses should be *controlled by the will* for a long lasting *healing effect.*
- Knowledge of these Yogic centres of Consciousness and its importance for mental relaxation is necessary for *Complete Health and Rehabilitation.*
  - *Sahasrara:* Centre of bliss purity and transparency.
  - *Ajna:* Centre for knowledge and wisdom that tranquilises the mind. A state of serenity always.
  - *Vishuddha:* Centre for selfless love. It strengthens Super ego-the ideal life principle.
  - *Anahat:* Centre of and for contentment. Emotional stability guides one's life smoothly. Modifies ego.
  - *Manipur:* Centre of activity, purpose in and for life. One can move in life, only if one wants to move.
  - *Swadhistana:* Centre for thinking. It is here where majority of us live, think, act, and behave. Personality of an individual shapes from here.
  - *Mooladhara:* Centre of one's original self. It is the demarcating centre between human nature and instinctive behaviour.

Our ancient healers understood only one concept of healing *"The Psychophysiological concept"*, hence the results were everlasting. As these chakras relate with human emotions, identifying the cause and effect of the disease and then concentrating and meditating on that chakra aids in the healing process of that diseased area.

"Chakras are more accurately, regions of mind power."

CHAKRAS: CENTRES OF HOMEOSTASIS

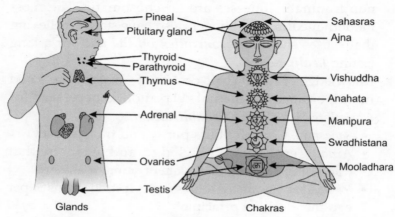

Pineal — Sahasras
Pituitary gland — Ajna
Thyroid
Parathyroid
Thymus — Vishuddha
— Anahata
Adrenal — Manipura
— Swadhistana
Ovaries — Mooladhara
Testis
Glands   Chakras

Fig. 7.5: Glands and Chakras—Centre of homeostasis

"In mutual collaboration with each each other, the endocrine glands and nervous plexuses maintain the internal enviroment of body leading to a state of physiological balance called as HOMEOSTASIS" (Fig. 7.5).

The Endocrine Glands:

- They form a wireless system.
- Hormones are secretions of these glands which are called as Chemical messengers.
- These glands are believed to have close relation with "chakras" that are responsible for maintaining internal environment of the body.

Nervous Plexuses:

- They form a wired system with all the nerves.
- These plexuses are thought to carry the currents of Pranic Energy as per Yogic texts.
- They are responsible for co-ordinating glandular functions.

The Homeostasis Effect

- The functioning of all vital signs of the body, i.e. Blood pressure, Heart rate, Respiratory rate and Temperature are under control of this "homeostasis effect".
- Yogic practice gives micro massage effect to these glands, reconditions these plexus thereby
  - improving vascularity and oxygenation
  - strengthening immunity.
- Yogic practice benefits directly the remotest areas of the body through the mediation of nervous plexus and indirectly through chemicals and endocrine mechanism in which the effects are felt more slowly.

"Meditating on these chakras as per their role performance harmonizes the external and internal environment, giving state of perfect health, tranquil mind and innate life style."

CHAKRAS AND FIVE COSMIC ELEMENTS

Table 7.1: Chakras and five cosmic elements

Chakras	Elements	Morale
Mooladhar	Earth	Be rooted to values in life.
Swadhisthana	Water	Flow with the current-flexibility.
Manipur	Fire	Keep the fire burning within-energy.
Anahat	Air	Open mindedness-spread fragrance.
Vishuddha	Ether	Accept life situation with smile.

SOME THOUGHTFUL ASPECTS ABOUT THESE CHAKRAS

1. Of the seven chakras, five are on the spine region signifying qualities of five cosmic elements: air, water, fire, earth and ether.
2. The *mooladhar* chakra is the foundation. It signifies how one is rooted to the ground. A firm foundation stabilizes the whole architecture.

3. Live in the present and always live with hope signifies the *mooladhar*.

4. One has to rise above the instinctive behaviour guides the *Swadhisthana* chakra.

5. The decision maker *Manipur* chakra, decides whether one wants to progress upwards or regress downwards towards worldly pleasures.

6. Over sensitivity can be a hindrance and lead to psychosomatic disease indicates the *Anahat* chakra.

7. Knowledge and foresight strengthen awareness encourages the *Vishuddha* chakra and the *Ajna* chakra respectively.

8. Chakras signify that man is complete within himself. Only thing is, one should identify, explore, cultivate and divert his potential towards Positive Creation and Well being.

The chakras encourage and enlighten that "Man is himself a complete universe."

Chapter 8

THE YOGIC PHYSIOTHERAPY

COMPARATIVE OUTLOOK: PHYSICAL EXERCISES AND YOGIC EXERCISES

Ideally speaking, Yogic practice should not be compared with any forms and types of exercises because Yogasanas and Pranayamas are not forms of exercises, though the primary component of both is *BODY* and primary goal of both is *POSITIVE HEALTH. Yogic exercises* lead to Complete Health, where in Physical Health is one of its aspects.

Life is not search for pleasure and perfection, but it is search for truth. Life is a continuous process. Things are happening so fast and change is inevitable. To cope up with this fast pace and a changing pattern, a state of alert but tranquilled mind is necessary. Happiness is within us only, why run around seeking for it outside.

The benefits of physical exercises are enormous and varied, *Yogic exercises are a special form of physical practice and performed through Asana (Yogic posture) and Pranayam (Yogic breathing).*

As many people worldwide are aware of Yogic practice, this comparative analysis is an effort just to strengthen their belief in these practices, with due faith and respect for physical exercises.

Table 8.1: The comparative guideline—physical exercise and yogic exercise

	Physiotherapy	Yogic Physiotherapy
	Physical exercises	*Yogic exercises*
1. Aim:	Physical Health	• Positive Health-comprising of Physical, Mental and Social and Spiritual.
2. Means:	Physiological Systems of body	• Through Psychophysiological systems of body.
3. Purpose:	Physical fitness and stability	• Self awareness and Harmony.
4. Posture:	Erect posture concept is its indicated factor.	• Erect posture concept-the key factor.
5. Target:	External Body: Body Structure and functions development and strengthening Attractive Personality.	• Internal Body: Strengthening and nourishing the mind and body. Pleasant Personality.
6. Outlook:	Conscious mind 10% of being/personality.	• Subconscious mind 90% of being/personality
7. Cultivates:	Begins with warming up and physical charging.	• Begins with prayers, mantra chanting and physical relaxation.
8.		
9.	Primary element is movement (slow or fast) hence effort required throughout physical performance.	• Primary element is an asana (relaxed posture) hence an effortless state of being and not doing.
10.	Concentrates more on muscular training through repetitive contractions	• Concentrates more on muscular relaxation through stretch stimulus facilitation.
11.	Energy expenditure and consumption due to physical performance, 3-14 cal/min.	• Energy conservation at all levels due to effortlessness, 0.8-3 cal/min.
12.	End results may be fatiguing as blood level of lactic acid concentration early and high.	• End result is relaxing and refreshing as negligible lactic acid concentrates in muscles.

Contd...

Contd...

	Physiotherapy	Yogic Physiotherapy
	Physical exercises	*Yogic exercises*
13.	Effects could be short lasting for overall performance..	• Effects long lasting for overall performance
14.	Open kinematics chain performance mostly favoring distal mobility	• Close kinematics chain performance for proximal stability (proximal stability must for distal mobility).
15.	Generally all physical fitness exercises focus on musculo-skeletal functioning with nervous system commands.	• They focus on all the internal systems, i.e. endocrines, nervous, digestive, cardio-respiratory which ultimately take care of musculoskeletal system.
16.	Effects: localized – physique.	• Effects: generalized & wholistic – Mind- body and soul.
17.	Personal benefits stressed as moral values, individual and social discipline if not indicated or encouraged.	• Generous, harmonizing benefits to one and all as the foundation of these exercises on Yam and Niyama.
18. *Physiological Effect:*	Increases muscular strength.	• Increases muscular relaxation and endurance.
19. *Purification Effect:*	Localized as per the type of exercises.	• Gross and generalized, as purifies all channels of body simultaneously.
20. *Therapeutic Effect:*	Specific effect on internal organs of body.	• Corrects functional disorders due to micro massage effect on internal oragns.

Contd...

Contd...

	Physiotherapy	Yogic Physiotherapy
	Physical exercises	*Yogic exercises*
21.	Overtraining can cause stress on these organs-lever, spleen, gallbladder.	• Regular practices strengthen these organs.
22. *Psychological Effect:*	Competitive spirit hence mind may be restless in some of the exercises.	• Content spirit hence mind relaxed, calm and tranquilled in all forms of practice.
23. *Psychosomatic Ailments:*	Limited Approach.	• An extensive positive approach for all psychosomatic ailments.
24. *Stress Coping Mechanisms:*	Physiological stresses may be overcomed.	• Psycho physiological stresses are overcomed.
25. *Immune System:*	Limited effect	• Strengthens, nourishes with definite effect.
26. *Economical Aspects*	Invasive, expensive package occasionally.	• Non-invasive, economical, no side effects, safe package always.
27. *Health Care Approach:*	Of Treating.	• Of Healing.
28. *Professionalism*	"A feeling of satisfaction."	• "A feeling of contentment."

Summary: The comparative guidelines quoted here are with respect and dignity to the physiotherapy profession that I belong to. The Yogic Physiotherapy mentioned is what I have experienced and fell during the course of my approach in Rehabilitation process.

THE INTEGRATED APPROACH— PHYSIO-YOGA

"When the senses are stilled, when the mind is at rest, when the intellect wavers not, and when the body is in perfect health – then say the wise, is reached the highest stage."
— Kathoupnishad.

YOGA IS BOTH A PHILOSOPHY AND TECHNOLOGY

- *Philosophy:* It guides us to what is the best objective in life. Its objective is "Positive health."
- *Technology:* It helps us to reach this objective. Its tools teachings, guidelines and ideology, present in scientific manner the effects it can have on human lifestyle. The Eight fold path of Ashtangyoga is an all embracing approach.
- The physiotherapist with the knowledge of basic science of Neuro-anatomy, Musculoskeletal physiology, Biomechanics, Sociology and Psychology can be an integral part of Rehabilitation team to assess the tools and techniques and thereby implement the guidelines and ideology of Ashtangyoga systematically, methodically and scientifically, I belive.

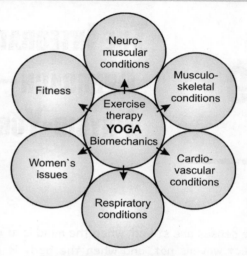

Disease Prevention and Cure

Fig. 9.1: The integrated approach

- The Yogic physiotherapy assessment and Ashtangyoga limbs approach can gain result which speaks for themselves for Rehabilitation in any Psychosomatic disorder or dysfunction.
- A brief explanation on both the approaches-Yogic and Physiotherapeutic based on my experience, analysis and feeling is quoted in the following manner:

Table 9.1: Yama and cone values

Yoga Philosophy	Physiotherapy
I. YAMA: Ethical discipline:	**CORE VALUES: For rapport building**
1. *Ahimsa:* Non violence in thought action and speech.	1. Compassion towards patients.
2. *Satya:* Truthfulness in thought, speech and action.	2. Honesty in practice.
3. *Asteya:* Non stealing.	3. Humility in patient's education.
4. *Brahmacharya:* Continence.	4. Devotion-practice in name of God.
5. *Aparigraha:* Non receiving	5. Dedication-selfless service.

Table 9.2: Niyama and Attitudes

II. NIYAMA: Observances:	ATTITUDE OF PATIENT: Understanding
1. *Saucha:* Purification.	1. Clarity in therapy.
2. *Santosh:* Contentment.	2. Fulfilment in approach.
3. *Tapas:* Austerity.	3. Sincerity in approach.
4. *Swadhayaya:* Self study.	4. Empathy.
5. *Ishwar pranidhan:* Surrender. to God.	5. Selflessness—Service to mankind is service to God.

- These two first steps of Ashtangyoga ladder of Yama and Niyama are foundation of Yoga and Physiotherapy practice.
- A healthy rapport develops between the patient and the professional, as the character of the healer is elevated and then aim becomes of giving rather than receiving.
- Ethical discipline and Observances of the patient, and Values and Attitudes of therapist yield positive results.

Table 9.3: Asana and Erect posture

III. ASANA: Yogic postures	Erect posture concept
1. Aim is to tone and tune the body to help the mind play the eternal symphony.	1. Aim is to strengthen the Postural mechanism for static and dynamic stability.
2. Brings consciousness from Subtle (soul) to Gross (body) harmonizing the whole human system by cellular activation.	2. Brings consciousness from Gross (body) to Subtle(soul) thus activating the whole psychophysiological system.
3. The three main types of Asanas incorporated are: • Meditative–Enlightenment (soul) • Relaxing–Relaxation(mind) • Cultural–Fitness (body)	3. The three fundamental postures focused in assessment • Lying–Righting reactions • Sitting–Protective reactions • Standing–Equilibrium reaction

- The physiotherapist may assess the need(mobility, strength, balance), modifies the posture guidance programme as per requirement and then educate the patient to follow the Yogic posture.

- These postures improve static and dynamic stability, reinforcing movements, as "proximal stability is must for distal mobility."
- The integration is of Position with Volition (movement with purpose).

Table 9.4: Pranayama and Breathing

IV. PRANAYAMA: Yogic breathing	Breathing patterns
1. Regulation of voluntary breath or bioenergy.	1. Normalise ventilation and facilitates respiration.
2. It cleanses and aeriate the lungs, oxygenate the blood, purifies the nerves.	2. Enhances thoracic mobility and expansion in all three directions. i.e. (a) vertical, (b) lateral (c) antero-posterior.
3. Conserves energy.	3. Channelizes the energy.
4. Significance of Kumbhaka-Breath control, is a facilitator of energy conservation.	4. Significance of diaphragmatic breathing is facilitator of ventilitatory function.
5. The effect is mainly on Immune system (endocrines, ANS) through mental relaxation.	5. The effect is mainly on cardio-respiratory system through physical relaxation.

- Analysing the respiratory mechanism, assessing the lung volumes and capacities by physiotherapist and, following the Yogic breathing techniques as per requirement replenishes and rejuvenates vigour and vitality improving overall function of the body.

Table 9.5: Pratyahara and Risk factor control

V. PRATYAHARA: Withdrawal of senses	Risk factor control
1. Inculcates social and individual discipline through mind control.	1. Inculcates physical discipline through body control.
2. Lifestyle modification through control of desires.	2. Lifestyle modification through code of conduct, sensible eating.

- The Yogic practice and physical application inhibits Tamas (Inertia), reduces Rajas (Hyperactivity) and increases Sattva (Harmony) gunas which give one a sense and feeling of well-being.

Table 9.6: Dharna and Volitional movement

VI. DHARNA: Concentration	Volitional movement
1. Pranayama silences the mind and Dharna is concentration on the silenced mind.	1. Patient participates into the movement performance (think into the movement).
2. Concentration leads to self determination and will power.	2. Volitional movement channelise and co-ordinate all systems of body improving postural stability and movement performance.

- Encouraging patient participation at all levels with guidance, motivation and breath regulation improve acceptance and tolerance of all situations, resulting in a flexible outlook and mobility.

Table 9.7: Dhyana and Balance and equilibrium

VII. DHYANA: Meditation	Balance and equilibrium
1. A continuous flow of positive energy.	1. A state of awareness—learning
2. A state of Attention (A-Tension).	2. A state of relaxation-physical.

- Mental concentration and attention improve physical balance and equilibrium always facililtating a state of relaxation (mental and physical) which improves task performances at all levels and in all situations (health or ill-health).

Table 9.8: Samadhi and Rehabilitation

VIII. SAMADHI: Illumination	Rehabilitation
1. Removes all obstacles with the above stated Yogic practice.	1. Integrates the person with the family, society and maintains the respect and dignity so that one can live a respectful life physically, mentally, socially and spiritually.

This experience of integrated approach has made me believe that every creature has as much right to live as he has. "I am born to help others and I should treat every person with care, comfort and compassion".

It has made me believe that my life is linked inextricably with those of others and has guided me to put the happiness of others before my own and to become a source of joy to all.

Section 2

Chapter 10

REHABILITATION— THE YOGIC WAY

"God Only Helps Them, Those Who Help Themselves"

Rehabilitation to me, as a Yoga student and as a Physical therapist, is identification, analysis and utilization of one's own existing immense capacities within oneself. This makes life more worthwhile and meaningful inspite of the disorder, dysfunction and disability.

REHABILITATION

- It has come from the latin word "Habil" which means "Able".
- The broadest and truest meaning is "return of ability".
- This word was first used by the church. The restoring of one's good name was called rehabilitation.
- It is a sense of restoration of good name, since it returns to the person respectability, acceptance and degree of social equality.
- Respect is always commanded and never demanded.
- The person who respects his or her own self, can respect any one, in any situation.
- "Principles of Yogic practice strengthen one's concept of "self" and encourage one to live with respect and dignity."

REHABILITATION: AS A YOGA DISCIPLE, MY INTERPRETATION OF THE 'WHO' (WORLD HEALTH ORGANIZATION) DEFINITION

It is a combined co-ordinated use of:

- **Social:** *Yama and Niyama* (Social and Individual discipline).
- **Medical:** *Asana and Pranayama* (Erect posture and Breath regulation).
- **Educational:** *Pratyahara,* (Risk factor control for prevention programme).
- **Vocational:** *Dharna and Dhyana* (Concentration and focused attitude in life) **training or retraining the individual for highest level of functional ability.**

"Self transformation leads to transformation of any situation".

THE NATIONAL COUNCIL OF REHABILITATION

- **Objectives:** To restore of an individual to his fullest social, economical, functional, psychological, emotional capability or usefulness.
- **Outlook:** Mental rehabilitation (personal dignity) facilitates Physical rehabilitation (body function restoration).
- **Application:** Cultivate, restore and conserve human resources with a multi disciplinary and multi dimensional concept.

"Yogic practice has a multi faceted approach for therapeutic results. The objective, outlook and applications, all are converged to "self".

Yoga believes that each individual has tremendous hidden resources within. What one needs to do is "spark the idea", and channelize the resources in right direction to recover faster from any illness or disease".

MEDICAL MODEL OF REHABILITATION AND YOGA

Here prevention is given the highest priority. It deals in five levels.

1. *Health Promotion:* This can be with health education, motivation and good nutrition which are adjusted to the various development phases of life and organizing of social and environmental conditions.

"Yoga also recommends for health promotion, moderation in lifestyle, food habits and behaviour patterns. It educates and encourages one, the importance of breath regulation to conserve energy. "Breath is the connecting link between mind and body."

"Healing the mind heals the body."

"Rehabilitating the mind rehabilitates the body."

2. *Specific protection:* This is prevention in its strictest sense. It suggests to identify the cause, reach to the grass root level of the disorder and get long lasting relief rather than treating the symptoms and getting immediate short lasting results.

"The Yogic concept of healing from within-without makes a person realize his or her own role as a cause, effect and outcome to manage all psychosomatic diseases, where the mind is the culprit and the body is the victim."

"Yogic practice improves acceptance and tolerance level."

3. *Early recognition and prompt treatment:* Its objective is to shorten the period of dysfunction.

"The spiritual tool of "self" in Yogic practice for early identification of the disease and intervention for regaining vigour and vitality concentrate on self introspection and self descipline. This definitely will enhance the recovery."

4. *Disability limitation:* The functional limitation may exist in any of the system dysfunction. It could be either due to Neuromuscular, Cardiovascular, Respiratory or Musculo skeletal disorders.

'The objective is to delay the consequences of clinical advancement of non preventable or non curative diseases.'

"Yoga helps in improving receptivity of subconscious mind, thereby strengthening the stress coping mechanism-mental and physical. This also leads to improved immunity."

The breath regulation techniques and short regular sessions of meditation help to deal with the demands of internal and external environment and personal needs, to create a state of psychological and physiological harmony.

5. *Rehabilitation:* This is more than just stopping the disease process.

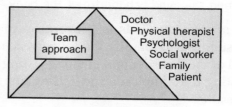

Fig. 10.1A: Medical rehabilitation

• Sometimes a feeling of dependency on support system.

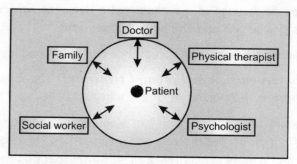

Fig. 10.1B: Yogic rehabilitation—my outlook

• Always a feeling of self worth and independence.

Rehabilitation is the primary and final goal of any therapy. Its objective is to restore **rights, privileges and reputation** of an individual. This could be for the Mental, Physical, Social, Vocational or Spiritual dimensions, or it could be as a part of therapeutic goal in dysfunctions of Neuromuscular conditions, Cardiovascular conditions, Respiratory conditions, Geriatric conditions or Musculoskeletal conditions.

- *Neuromuscular rehabilitation:* Pranayama, Meditation and Asanas.
- *Musculoskeletal rehabilitation:* Asana, Pranayama and Meditation.
- *Respiratory rehabilitation:* Pranayama, Pratyahaar (life style modification), Meditation.
- *Cardiovascular rehabilitation:* Niyama, Pratyahaar, Pranayama and Meditation.

All the professionals involved in rehabilitation should walk along with the patient, on the path of healing and recovery, rather than just giving instructions, prescriptions and treatment applications. This is the Yogic principle for Rehabilitation.

SUMMARY

- The secret of rehabilitation is to give right help at right time.
- Psychological and Social adjustment begin early in rehabilitation.
- Emotional and Mental attitudes can have a decisive effect on the outcome of rehabilitation process.
- It is quoted that rehabilitation is the third phase, after preventive and curative aspects of medical care.
- **My experience with Yoga has given direction to my thoughts and strengthened my belief that "Mental**

rehabilitation" is in fact the first step in medical care for prevention and cure of any diseases.

- Rehabilitation team experts can guide, motivate, support, help but ultimately it is the person himself or herself who has to take charge of his or her own life to respond effectively to the rehabilitation programme.

- I firmly believe that if a person is emotionally balanced, mentally capable , strong and determined he can take care of his physical health irrespective of any illness or disease.

- "Yoga—an easy, economical, enriching and empowering success key for rehabilitation, which can be practised by all, is associated with universal laws for respect of life, truth and patience, thereby improving the quality of life."

Chapter 11

APPLICATIONS OF YOGA

"There is definite connection between Mental agility and Physical vitality. Physical transformation in vibrancy, energy and enthusiasm depends on Mental fitness".

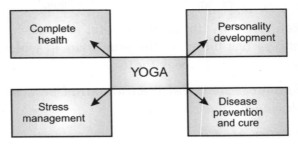

Fig. 11.1: Applications of yoga

- As a well cut diamond having many sides and projections, each of which illuminate a different colour of light, my experience with Yoga encourages me to understand each aspect deeply and to make an effort to apply its rays of light to bring about a quality transformational change within *"self"* of each person to prevent him from getting affected by the modern day life stresses.
- This amazing science has motivated me to first inculcate within me and then apply the morale of the first seven steps of Ashtanyoga in the therapeutic programme as per the goals targeted for the *Rehabilitation*.

"Yoga is associated with universal laws for respect of life with patience, persistence, perseverence, practice and positivism to improve the quality of life."

THE APPLICATIONS

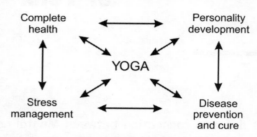

Fig. 11.2: The Inter-relationships of Yoga Applications

"Yoga is each time and every movement a living act."

With reference to the above quote, and based on my experience; I feel these are the *four areas* in which, Yogic practice and its result speak for itself.

All four areas are *interdependent, intradependent* but are still *independent* of each other.

The four areas are :-

1. Personality Development.

2. Stress Management.

3. Complete Health.

4. Disease Prevention and Cure.

It is beyond the capacity of this book to explain all four dimensions' application. The focus being in this book is on "Complete health" and "Disease prevention and cure".

1. Personality Development

"One should have a personality as gentle as a dove and as strong as a lion".

— Quotable quote.

- *"Persona"* means *"mask"*.
- Personality is Ego consciousness, not Ego in terms of inflated pride, but a consciousness of **"I Exist"**.
- *It is a monotonous way of thinking, feeling and behaving of an individual.*
- Personality of an individual can be influenced by *three dimensions*, as per the psycho analysts. These influences are:
  - Genetic influences.
  - Environmental influences.
  - Integrated Ego, i.e. "I Exist."
- Balance of the three dimensions of *Cognition (knowledge), Conation (Character)and Affect (Emotion)* is personality development.
- *"Yoga* believes that personality of an individual can be developed not just by *Ego strengthening but by 'Ego purification'."*
- This "Ego purification" can be achieved by "Ashtangyoga ladder":
  - Yama and Niyama **develop character** of an individual.
  - Asanas **develop the external self** of a person.
  - Pranayama **regulates this external self with the character** of an individual.
  - Pratyahaar makes a person **aware about his code of conduct in life**.
  - Dharna **enhances him towards a focused life**.
  - Dhyana **harmonizes an individual's internal self with his external self**.

"One can be whatever one wants to be with a spiritual outlook and concentration in life".

2. Stress Management

"Stress is essential in life and for life".

What is stress???

The way our mind and body respond to the damaging and harmful situation, which arise due to change in our environment (mental and physical) for adjustment is stress.

- Severity of stress depends on *"stressors"* which depends on individual's perception of stress and stressors.

- There could be *physical stressors (like heat, cold, noise and illness), family stressors, environmental stressors, interpersonal stressors, carrier and job related stressors and economical stressors.*

- *Eu-stress* is successful handling of stress which is dependent on one's *own stress coping mechanism.*

- **Stress management** understands the demand (stressors) of the situation, perceives it as a part of life and its growth, thereby making adjustments within self and surroundings.

- *Yoga practice of* :
    - Yama and Niyama *reduces inter personal relationship and social stress.*
    - Asanas and Pranayama *reduce physical and mental stress.*
    - Pratyahara manages stress by *withdrawal from desires* through adjustment in beliefs and attitudes.
    - Dharna helps in *organizing and improving tolerance level.*
    - Dhyana *strengthens the* Stress coping mechanism.

3. Complete Health

Positive health and Complete health are almost same as per my view and thinking.

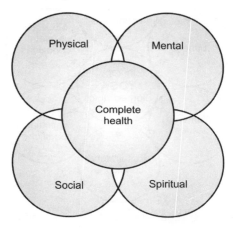

Fig. 11.3: Complete health

- *Yoga* analysts explain HEALTH as *"the moral manifestation of life force under favorable environment, creating perfect harmony with them and obeying the laws that govern them, is the state which is ordinarily understood by the common expression "health".*
- The Complete health of an individual depends upon the quality and quantity of his PRANA-The life force.
- The life force in every individual is his healing power.
- *All four* aspects have a mutual responsibility and equal duty to be performed for maintaining Complete health, i.e. *Physical, Mental, Social and Spiritual.*
- One can understand from the **Fig. 11.3** that for complete health, *emotions need to be calm, cool, and balanced.* All four aspects function effectively with healthy *Emotional Quotient.*

"Yoga chittavritti nirodh"-training the mind trains the body."
— Patanjali

4. Disease Prevention and Cure

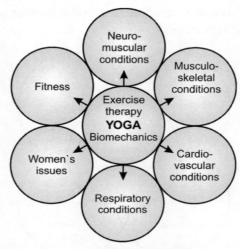

Fig. 11.4: Yoga—disease prevention and cure

"Health means the life under natural conditions, where the laws of adaptation and other laws that govern the environment are not violated in the least." If the laws are violated, if the condition be abnormal, and if adaptation be imperfect, then the result will be *"a state of ill health."*
- *If the PRANA-the life force fails to attack the enemy, defend or protect, then the result will be disease.*
- To apply the principles and techniques, it is necessary to review some of its *objectives* that can be implemented for *Rehabilitation.*

The objectives of Yoga in disease prevention and cure:
1. *Non attachment* towards all worldly material things that are pain causing **(Yama and Niyama).**
2. *Self Purification:* To be fearless and truthful always. Fear grips a man and makes him paralyzed. Freedom from fear comes only to those who lead a pure life. One should not fear about future consequences of disease **(Yama, Niyama, Asana, Pranayama).**

3. *Self Realization:* A "Realized self" can conquer all battles and sufferings. One should fight all battles with love. Gentleness of mind is its main attribute. One should accept the fact that it is one's own self that has caused the disease, and it is this self only which will heal **(Pratyahara, Dharna)**.

4. *Self Actualization:* Meditation, listen to the signals and commands of body with honesty, sincerity and love, and then finally leave it to GOD. A feeling of surrender helps in recuperating faster from illness.

"Yoga is not a means for disease cure, but a 'realised self' can prevent and help in recovering from the consequences of the disease".

• In this section my request to all the readers, is to read the chapters with a sensitive, illogical, irrational and non-analytical mind some of the creative charateristic of the right brain and make an effort to try and practise on oneself first and then to apply for any **Rehabilitation** purpose.

• The expression put forward in these chapters is based on what I have studied and on the inspirations from the teachings of all my teachers of Physiotherapy and Yoga and last but not the least from *my patients' faith and students' trust in me*.

"The effort is not to prove but is to share my experience of learning and its application with an integrated approach."

YOGA AND BIOMECHANICS

"Qualities of self reliance, self esteem and independence are achieved by emotional maturity; through awakening the hidden potential energy within one's own body."

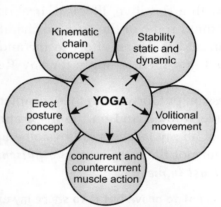

Fig. 12.1: Yoga and principles of biomechanics

"A firm foundation is must for a house to stand." The qualities further more required are discipline faith, tenacity and perseverance.

For enhancing improvement in postural control and balance training, kinesthetic sense is essential. Principles of Biomechanics and its application can facilitate this sense. It is an essential element for the comprehensive *Rehabilitation* of the patient.

BIOMECHANICS

- Broadly defined as science of *human motion.*
- The application of mechanics to living human body is *biomechanics.*
- This science hence requires theories and principles from Anatomy, Physiology, Psychology and Mechanics.
- The basic kinesiology is concerned with normal and intact *Neuromuscular, Musculoskeletal systems* with normal *Psyche.*
- The purpose of understanding biomechanics is to apply its principles in management procedures so that human performance may be improved.
- The clinical applications of biomechanics meet the needs in the field of rehabilitation of many *Psychosomatic ailments.*

YOGIC PRACTICE

- Broadly defined as science of supreme *harmonization of body, mind and soul.*
- The application of "**Concept of Self**" in body functioning is *Yoga.*
- This science hence requires theories and principles that maintain a *stable body, regulated breath and tranquil mind.*
- The purpose of understanding Yogic science is to apply its principles to *replenish, rejuvenate and reorganize* oneself for rehabilitation.

THE INTEGERATED APPROACH

Table 12.1: Biomechanics and yogic practice

Biomechanics	Yogic science
Physical aspect: Balance the body based on mechanics and its application. **Indications:** • Economy of effort • Avoidance of injury • Improvement of performance	**Psychological aspect:** Balancing the body through balancing the emotion. **Indications:** • Energy conservation • Relaxation: mental and physical • A sense of well being

The Biomechanical Assessment

   I. Erect Posture Concept.
  II. Static and Dynamic Stability Components.
 III. Joint Dynamics – Open Kinematic and Close Kinematics.
 IV. Movement Patterns – Voluntary and Volitional.
  V. Muscle Dynamics – Concurrent and Countercurrent Action.

The Yogic Practice

- The *Ashtangyoga ladder* can be explained with reference to above biomechanical factors.
- *Yama, Niyama and Pratyahara* are foundation pillars for stability.
- *Asanas* for Static Stability and Erect Posture Concept.
- *Pranayama* for Dynamic Stability.
- *Dharna and Dhyana* for Energy Conservation.
- *YOGA* brings alignment between the two halves of body and finer adjustments within body components.
- *In Yogic Posture,* the Stretch Effect from toes to top of the head in defiance of gravity strengthens *the Postural Mechanisms* thoroughly.

"Yoga converts human potential energy into kinetic energy"

WHAT IS HUMAN POTENTIAL ENERGY IN YOGA

- *Energy* is capacity of body.
- *Potential Energy* is the capacity of the body of doing work by virtue of its position.
- *Kinetic Energy* is body's capacity of doing work because of its velocity.
- Our body has great energy feeling within. It just needs to be reactivated. This can only be possible with inclusion of higher levels of thinking namely *"Ego and Intellect."*
- The main energy source and drive lies in the *emotional system* in the brain and this is in *Hypothalamus*. This energy is responsible for emotions like *love, hatred, fear, anger, hunger control, thirst and sex drive* believes Yoga science. Whereas modern science believes that energy generation in brain is through *electro chemical process.*
- It is important to understand this energy. It is this energy which gives person a healthy disease free life.
- Yoga practice helps to channelise this potential energy for biomechanical function of Activities of Daily Living.
- Yoga believes that this energy in its potential form is at the level of base of *sacral spine.*
- Yoga believes that this Potential energy can be converted to Kinetic form either *spontaneously or by Meditational practice.*

1. ERECT POSTURE

The Biomechanical View

- Movement begins and ends in a posture. Posture follows a movement like a shadow.
- There are innumerable concepts of human postures and innumerable interpretations of its symptoms.

- Posture to a physiotherapist is a gauge of:
  - Mechanical Efficiency
  - Kinesthetic Sense
  - Joint Mobility
  - Muscle Balance
  - Neuromuscular Coordination
  - Habitual Carriage
  - Stress Coping Mechanism
  - Balance of vital organs function of Respiration, Circulation, Digestion and Elimation.

Newton's Laws and Postural Mechanism

The force of gravity acts continuously on human body and if unopposed, the latter will fall to the ground. This effect of gravity can be counteracted by a force equal in its *magnitude, direction, and point of application,* that is, Antigravitational force. The Antigravitational forces are dependent on the Postural mechanisms comprising of *antigravity mechanisms, postural fixation, counterpoising mechan-isms,righting reactions, tilt reactions, protective reactions and equilibrium reactions.* Only when the mind and body complex work in synchrony and harmony, the volitional act of postural mechanism can be responsible for erect posture.

Erect Posture: The Yogic View

- Yoga calls it as an **Asana - *The Yogic Posture.***
- It is a *state of being* and not doing. This is an *effortlessness* state where the mind is concentrated on *Infinity* and with a sense of *bliss.*
- The channelization of the potential energy can only be possible with an erect posture.
- All Asana emphasize on Erect Spine Concept, whether in sitting or standing.
- Each Yogic posture has *physical, mental, health and spiritual benefits.*

- The standing poses signify all aspects of Erect Spine Concepts. *Strength of Yoga lies in these poses.*
- They *stretch, strengthen, tone and activate* all the different joints and parts of body.
- They *realign* the complete anatomy while removing muscular imbalances.
- They prepare for all other asanas in forward, backward, sideward bends and twists.

Tadasana: For Erect Posture

- *Tada* means *mountain*, that signifies steadiness, straight, upright and unmoved.
- It is the *foundation* for all standing Asana.

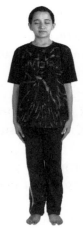

Fig. 12.2: Tadasana—the erect posture

- It is a pose that implies *firmness* of erect posture.
- It helps to teach correct standing thereby with regular practice it improves posture of individual.
- We spend hours standing but never realize or never give a thought as to whether we stand correctly.

Technique—Tadasana

- *Stand erect* with feet together, heels and big toes next to each other, rest the heels and metatarsals on the floor and stretch all the toes flat on floor.
- *Tighten* the knees and pull the kneecaps (patella) up.
- *Contract* the hip muscles and pull it up together (Glutii).
- Keep the stomach in, chest forward, spine stretched and neck straightened.
- Distribute the body weight evenly on both the feet.
- For convenience one can place the arms by the side of thighs.

Advantages

- *Symmetrical weight bearing* on both feet and effortless hold.
- Body feels *light, energetic and acquires agility.*
- *Strengthen*s all antigravity musculature.

Pathomechanics

- If weight unevenly distributed on both legs, spinal deviations and deformities result *hampering spinal soft tissues elasticity.*
- Heels and toes if not in line parallel to median plane, develop *tightness in flexors and adductor group of muscles of hip.*
- If weight more on heels than, posterior tilting of pelvis, *abdomen protrudes, swayback* and back problems result.

It is pre-requisite to encourage the art of correct standing than go on stressing and elaborating on back strengthening exercise programme.

An erect standing posture is a co-ordinated framework of supple body, regulated breath, relaxed mind, appropriate extero-receptive and intero-receptive sensory input.

Pranayama for Erect Posture

Anulom – Vilom (Alternate nostril breathing) for relaxed posture.

- Skeletal muscles also work for long periods of time without fatigue, provided their contraction alternates regularly with complete relaxation. *Consequent* replenishment of the blood supply bring oxygen to repair the effects of continuous standing and remove metabolic products.

- Postural muscles cannot be relaxed completely when involved at work, but *replenishment of oxygen* can be maintained continuously by regular practise of pranayama, as it reduces oxygen consumption of muscles, avoids muscles fatigue, aids repair and removes, wastes.

Yogic breathing facilitates strengtheing of postural mechanisms

II. STATIC AND DYNAMIC STABILITY

The Biomechanical View

- *Static Stability:* Centre of body must project within the base of support, e.g. standing and sitting.

- *Dynamic Stability:* Centre of gravity of body must project within the base of support with changing position of body movements and centre of gravity. It is brought about by the co-ordinated effort of bony structures, ligaments, muscle co-ordination and most importantly "**The Psyche State.**"

- This stability is maintained by body adjustments as per say, and applied in all activities of daily living to overcome stress.

- *Fixation and Stability:* Purpose of both is same, to *strengthen stability component, i.e. the non-rotatory horizontal component of muscle.*

- *Fixation* describes *state of immobility* brought about by co-contraction of muscles.

- *Stabilization* is state of relative immobility.

- Exercises done more slowly require greater muscular effort and control and strengthen the stability component of muscle.

- *Eccentric contraction* of muscles aids to strengthen the stability component of muscles.

"For rehabilitation of patient or in conditioning programme one cannot use either of the two exclusively. A combination of both (stability and mobility components of muscles) is required for functional tasks."

Static and Dynamic Stability: The Yogic View

- *Balance and Harmony* of body is brought about by *balanced mind and regulated breath.*

- Breath is the connecting link between mind and body.

- Stability: Static and dynamic both are dependent on emotional poise and balance.

- Pranayama is an essential mode to achieve this state.

- This state is further strengthend *in Yogic posture* (Asana) which are set to be *Psychophysical posture.*

- Asana: Dynamic state – process of *going into* and *releasing out* of state of Asana.

- Asana: Static state – The Yogic posture itself.

Ushtrasana: The Camel Posture

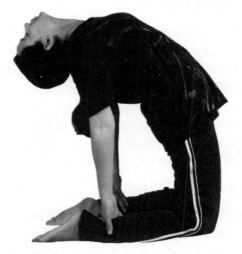

Fig. 12.3: Ushtrasana—An asana of static and dynamic stability

Technique: Ushtrasana

- Kneel on the floor, with knees and ankles together and toes flat with soles upturned.
- Bend backwards and grasp the ankles.
- Extend the head backward and arch the spine pushing pelvis forward.
- Breathe freely and maintain the pose.
- Hold for fifteen to thirty seconds as per comfort (static stability).
- Release the pose gradually (dynamic stability).
- Kneel, sit and gradually return to starting position.
- Place hands with palms turned on lap.
- Relax for few seconds.

Biomechanical Analysis of Ushtrasana (As Dynamic Stable Posture)

- *Wide base* of support.
- Low centre of gravity.
- Line of centre of gravity *within* the base of support.
- With full *chest expansion* and lung capacity the *stability increases.*
- All segments of body balance each other (Segmentation).
- *Eyes closed*, so mind *concentrated within* (Psychophysical).
- *Balanced mind leads to balanced stable posture.*

Advantages

- *Co-contraction* of all spinal muscles. This when *released increases vascularity* to all tissues (Reactive hyperaemia).
- *Strengthens* the Extensors of spine and stretches all anterior structures.
- *Stretch Reflex Facilitation* thereby improving contractile ability of Abdominals.
- Shoulders Extended and externally rotated, Scapula retracted, *corrects Drooping shoulder postures.*
- *Micro massage* effect to all abdominal organs and pelvic viscera.

"Quietness and calmness of mind come with regulated breath aiding stability—static and dynamic."

III. KINEMATIC CHAIN CONCEPTS

- In rehabilitation literature and biomechanics application, human motions or exercise are often described or classified as occurring in *"open" or "closed"* pattern.
- Kinematic describes sciences of motion of body in space and forces that cause this movement.
- *Kinetic:* Movement of a body.
- *Kinematic:* Muscular forces of a body.

Kinematic Chain: Biomechanical Analysis

- *Open kinematic chain* exercise mainly *facilitates* the *Vertical* movement component of muscles.
- Open kinematic facilitates *angular* movements of joints and *asscessory* movements too.
- Individual *isolated muscle group* strengthen with open kinematic through stimulation of muscle proprioceptors.
- *Close kinematic chain* exercise facilitates the non rotatory stability component of muscles.
- Close kinematic is *more functional chain* of movements in ADL.
- They *improve power, strength and endurance* simultaneously thereby reducing functional limitations at a time and improve physical performance.
- *Joint proprioceptors* are stimulated through approximation in close kinematic chain which increases *stabilization* factor thoroughly.
- Joint and muscle mechanoreceptors are also stimulated, are favoring co-contraction of Agonists and Antagonists which subsequently promote Dynamic Stability.

Kinematic Chain: Yogic View

- *Yogic postures* along with *Yogic breath control, Concentration and Contemplation* (meditation) fulfills and justify both the aspects of kinematic chains thereby aiding the rehabilitation programme easily.

Sarpasana

Technique

- Lie flat on abdomen, leg stretched and together, soles of feet turned up.
- Place the hands flat on floor against the side of the waist of body, fingers pointing forward, elbow bent.
- Chin rested down on floor.

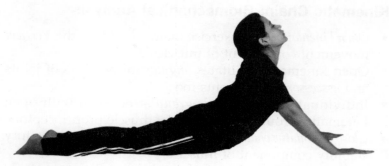

Fig. 12.4: Sarpasana—An asana of close kinematic chain pattern - UL

- While inhaling slowly raise the head, neck and upper back taking weight on hands. Rise till chest off the floor (Bhujangasana) Sarpasana-rise till umbilical level with elbow extended.
- Hold the pose for 15 to 30 seconds, release the pose gradually exhaling slowly through nose.

Advantages

- A *Close kinematic chain* exercise and posture for the *upper component of body* and back as the distal segments of upper limbs fixed.
- *Strengthens* the anti gravity components of *Trapezius, Rhomboids, Thorasic and Lumber Extensors.*
- Co-contraction of Protractors and Retractors of Scapula *prevents Shoulder Arm Complex and Cervical Spine Painful Syndromes.*
- The extended spine position and release, *recondition the spinal nerves* functioning by increased vascularity.
- Intra-abdominal and pelvic pressure increases *improved Glandular* functions in that area, thereby giving vigour and vitality.
- This postures are performed with mind body concentration hence *Psychophysical* benefit both are achieved.

INTEGRATED CONCEPT OF KINEMATIC CHAIN

Table 12.2: Principles of biomechanics of yoga

Open Kinematic Chain	Close Kinematic Chain
• Distal segments *move* in space.	• Distal segments remain *stationary*.
• Joint movements are *independent*.	• Joint movements are *inter dependent*.
• May or may *not* be Mass movement activity.	• *A Mass movement pattern* activity.
• Muscle work facilitates *Prime movers*.	• Muscles facilitated are *Proximal Stabilizers*.
• Asana: *Going into and out of the posture*.	• *The Asana itself*.
• May or may not require a Psychophysical movement.	• The pattern of position controlled Psychophysically.
• Used for *Exercise training* programme.	• Used for *Functional re-eduction* programme.

IV. MOVEMENT CONCEPT

- It is a fundamental characteristic of all animal life, and means by which the organism adapts itself to the demands made upon it by the environment in which it lives.
- Under normal conditions a single muscle never works alone to produce a movement or secure stability. Functionally muscles work in groups, i.e. Antagonists, Agonists, Synergists, Fixators, etc.

Movement Facilitation; Biomechanical View

- *"Proximal stability is must for distal mobility and skill."*
- Movements can be classified as *Voluntary, Volitional and Ballistic* when performed actively.
- Voluntary movement is initiated in response to demand made by sensory stimulation.
- Magnitude of force relative to magnitude of résistance is decisive factor to cause motion.

Movement Facilitation: Yogic View

- Yogic posture (Asana) is a combined act of voluntary, volitional and ballistic movements.
- Yogic breathing (Pranayama) co-ordinates the mental movements (thoughts) and physical movements, facilitating movement performance.

Paschimottanasana

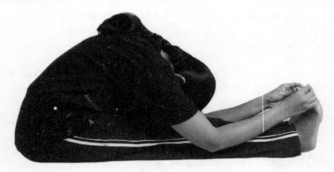

Fig. 12.5: Paschimottanasana—movement facilitation

- *Paschim* means *West*. Back of the body is West according to Yogic science. Front of the body is East, Head is North and Soles are South.
- In this pose, posterior aspect of the body, i.e. Paschim is extensively and completely stretched, hence the name.
- This extensive stretch, *stimulates the stretch receptors* facilitating strength of anti-gravity muscles.

Advantages

- *Improves digestion, corrects constipation, eliminates wastes* due to the squeezing and micro massage effect on abdominal organs.
- *Slims the waist and makes body symmetric, well built and supple* by selective stretching of hamstrings and waist muscles.

- *Reconditioning of spinal nerves* through this posture as increased vascularity.
- Helps mind to attain qualities of concentration and relaxation improving movement performance.
- Facilitates the process into Meditation.
- Controls and regulates sexual urges.

"Yogasanas are more Volutional Movement Performance achieving Ballistic Scale and Strengthening Reflex Activity."

CONCURRENT AND COUNTERCURRENT MUSCLE DYNAMICS

- The two joint Tendon action of muscle obeys the principle of Length-Tension Relationships.
- The efficiency of a two joint muscle is substantially influenced by position of two joints.

Biomechanical View

- Favourable length tension relationships are maintained by movement combinations whereby the muscle is elongated by movement at one joint while producing force at another joint.
- The Rectus femoris is more efficient as knee extensor if hip extends simultaneously with knee (Prone SLR).
- The Hamstrings are more efficient as hip extensors when knee extend simultaneously (Countercurrent action).
- The Rectus Femoris can perform hip flexion more effectively if knee flexes simultaneously with hip because it favours muscle to contract within favorable range (Concurrent action).

Yogic View

- Yogic postures like Naukasana (Nauka-boat) strengthen the anti-gravity mechanism through stretch-stimulus effect, proprioceptive stimulation and muscle co-contraction.
- These psychophysical postures regulate the breath and improve concentration.

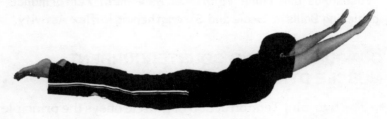

(A) Naukasana—The boat pose (prone)

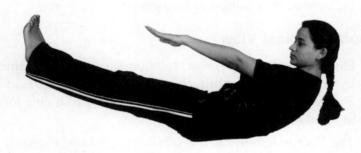

(B) Naukasana—The boat pose (supine)

Figs 12.6A and B: Muscle length—Tension relationship

- Both these Asanas are complementary postures to each other.
- They improve static stability of spine and dynamic stability of lower limb musculature through this length – tension relationship of Hamstrings and Rectus Femoris.

Advantages

- It also favors principles of *Reciprocal Relaxation*.
- Very useful Asana for women with *Menorrhagia and Menopause.*

SUMMARY: YOGA AND BIOMECHANICS

Table 12.3: Yoga and Biomechanics

Biomechanics' Principles and Yoga:

• The Erect Posture	*Asanas*	• The Anti-gravity Mechanisms
• Static and Dynamic Stability	*Asanas and Pranayama*	• Co-contraction
• Kinematic Chain Concept	*Asanas and Pranayamas*	• Stabilizing
• Movement Facilitation	*Asanas and Pranayamas*	• Mechanisms
• Length-Tension Relationship	*Asanas*	• Psychophysical Application
		• Two-Joint Tendon Action

YOGA AND EXERCISE THERAPY

"The Tension of the muscles can be affected by conscious thought and effort, and can be relieved by the application of conscious thought or muscular effort on the part of a person "(Mind Body Concept)."

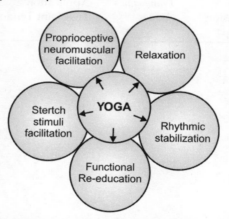

Fig. 13.1: Yoga and its applications in exercise therapy

- The word 'Exercise': 'Ex' means 'out', 'Erc' means 'to lock'. Hence exercise means 'to unlock' the body and make it free to move.
- The word 'Yoga' means 'to join,' 'to unite,' 'to connect' the mind and body.

- The word 'Therapy' means 'to heal,' 'to treat,' 'to care and correct'.

"The combination of YOGA and EXERCISE according to me, is that, its only when the mind connects in totality with body, in thoughts, speech and actions, the body can unlock itself to function freely in life to achieve positive health. Understanding the principles of both the sciences and its applications for therapeutic purpose yields comprehensive care and 'Rehabilitation' of a person."

Exercise Therapy Aims To

1. **Explain** the role and need of exercise to the patient.
2. **Demonstrate** the exercise to be practised and then perform.
3. **Focus** on the quality of exercise performance is important than quantity (Repetitions).
4. **Choose** the exercise schedule as per patient's clinical capacity.
5. **Modify the progress** of exercise only after regular assessment.
6. **Prescribe exercise** on biomechanical principles for productive results.
7. **Prescribe exercise** on fundamental patterns for better outcome.
8. **Ensure** 'Rest' in between the sessions to overcome *overuse and overstrain*.

Yogic Practice Aims To

1. **Replenish** energy stores.
2. **Remove** physiological and metabolic wastes from blood and body tissues.
3. **Replenish** oxygen reserves in the tissues.

4. **Rejuvenate** with abundant supply of oxygen for aiding muscle relaxation.
5. **Recharge** patient's Attention, Motivation and Feedback for influencing patient's performance in exercise programme.
6. **Restore** a sense of well-being by dynamic activity facilitation.
7. **Regulate** Exercise programmed Breath regulation.
8. **Rehabilitate** the physical, mental, social and spiritual aspect of a person.

TYPES OF EXERCISES AND YOGIC APPLICATION

1. *Active Exercises:* The slow rhythmic movement to go into a state of Asana and release the state of Asana is an active process. The exercise performed is completely at a person's will. *The Yogic exercises also comprise of Psychophysical performance.*
2. *Hold-Relax:* "The Yogic posture held." The longer the hold, greater is the relaxation. *Greater the mind relaxation and breath control, greater the hold and greater the relaxation.*
3. *Stretching Exercises:* An End range hold in Asanas physiologically improves soft tissue pliability especially of ligaments and muscles.
4. *Joint Mobilization Techniques:* The "*Sukshma Kriyas*" also known as Yogic warm ups facilitate accessory movements of **glide and roll** of the joints for effective full range of angular motion of joint.
5. *Resisted Exercises:* These exercises increase power, physical strength and endurance. **Yogic practice overcomes mental resistance and improves functional strength** which relates to ability of the neuromuscular system to produce, reduce, or control forces as per the demand of the situation for better effective long lasting performance of the task.

6. *Agility Exercises:* Yogic warm ups and *"The Surya-namaskar Cycle"* when practised with breath regulation fulfills more effectively the goals of agility exercises (The fast cycle).

7. *Relaxation Exercise:* The ultimate goal of Yogic practice is Mind Body Relaxation and **Energy conservation to meet** the challenges of life situation with vigour and vitality.

8. *Breathing Exercises:* Yoga believes in regulation of mind through breath regulation. Breath is the link **between mind and body.** The foundation of physical health is regulated breath. **"The Yogic breathing is the soul of Yoga science."**

9. *Co-ordination Exercise:* The Raj-Yoga ladder of sage Patanjali, to be followed for internal and external harmony and to be in a state of balance and poise physically, mentally and socially. 'The concept of "Self" **leads one to be well organised being.**

10. *Aerobic Exercises:* Low intensity repetitive total body movements like walking, jogging, swimming improves oxygen uptake by the body and improves cardio pulmonary endurance. **The Suryanamaskar Cycle fulfills the goal.**

11. *Strengthening Exercises:* To improve strength, power, endurance and functional capacity by different methods and application. **The Yogic practise of Asana fulfills all the principles of strengthening.**

12. *Postural and Balance Exercises:* The Raj-Yoga ladder: The first two steps of **Yama and Niyama** make a firm foundation for an erect posture. **Asana** strengthens the postural muscles. **Pranayama** improves respiratory muscle's tone. **Pratyahara** prevents mind and muscle fatigue. **Dharna** improves stability through concentration and **Dhyana**-Meditation achieves the balance. (Mental and Physical)

Table 13.1: Yogasana: An all in one package

- Active exercises.
- Hold and relax.
- Stretching exercises.
- Strengthening exercises.
- Mobility exercise.
- Agility exercises.
- Resisted exercises.
- Relaxation exercises.
- Breathing exercises.
- Co-ordination exercises.
- Aerobic exercises.
- Postural exercises.

PRINCIPLES OF EXERCISE THERAPY AND YOGIC APPLICATION

1. *Hook's Law:* Strain is directly proportional to applied Stress.

   Yogic postures are psychophysical posture. They are based on Self analysis and self prescription pattern. A stress free mind leads to strain free muscles, which can improve the quality of muscle dynamics and hence improve functional mobility.

2. *Principle of Elastic behaviour of Material:* Uttanasan

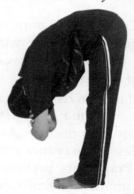

Fig. 13.2: Uttanasana—Principle of elastic behaviour of material

When material is stressed within its elastic phase, the strain or deformation which occurs is reversible. The material will return to its original length and shape. This is the region in which it is safe to stress most materials without damage occurring.

Yogasana and Pranayama are Self management exercise as one is constantly watching, guiding and controlling the rhythm of contraction. The Yogic posture includes this aspect of physiological lengthening or extensibility of soft tissue around the joints which can prevent and overcome continuous loading stress and strain on activities of daily living.

3. *Relaxation:* Volumes have been written by health professionals of many disciplines on relaxation training methods and application. Relaxation as a means of exercise therapy helps to integrate general relaxation procedures into an intervention programme to improve mobility. Massage, Biofeedback, Neuromuscular facilitation techniques, Progressive Muscular Relaxation Technique and Hydrotherapy are some means.

"Yogic practise regularly relaxes the mind, which recuperates the nerve centres in the body and revitalize and invigorates so that body gets recharged."

Technique of Relaxation: Egyptian Pose

- It is the most simple, practical easy posture.
- It is also called as "Chair posture."
- Sit on a straight back chair, head and spine in vertical line.
- The knees and feet together with thighs resting on chair's seat.
- The palms kept resting on the thighs.

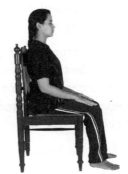

Fig. 13.3: The chair pose— Principle of relaxation

- The feet resting on the floor.
- Breathe freely.
- Eyes closed.

Advantages

- This posture can be assumed by patients having back and knee arthritis.
- It also provides the sitting position for practising Pranayama and Meditation too.
- Every opportunity should be taken to sit for several minutes in this posture, watching television, listening to the music and in conversation.

4. *"The tension in the muscles is generated by tension in thought processes."* This concept is accepted worldwide today. May it be in field of Sports, Technology, Business, Education, Research, etc. Less Stress response is evident in Creative people research states. If body is only considered then why the difference?

"Relaxed Mind Leads To Relaxed Body."

- Physiological Relaxation could be achieved by two methods
  - *Contrast Method:* Strong contraction of a muscle followed by Relaxation of the same muscle.
  - *Reciprocal Method:* Contraction of agonist relaxes the antagonists.

Yogic postures fulfill both the principle of physiological relaxation simultaneously. In the "state of Asana" the muscles that are contracted to hold the Asana, give reciprocal relaxation to the antagonists of the hold. And when the "hold" is released the same muscles relax reciprocally (Agonists).

- Continuity and a sense of universality comes in a knowledge of the inevitable alteration of tension and relaxation in the internal rhythms of which each inhalation and exhalation constitutes with one cycle wave or vibration with Pranayama.

"Yogic breathing, concentration methods and meditation are also great means of achieving relaxation".

5. *Stretch reflex and reciprocal relaxation:*
    - Stretch reflex can be used to obtain lengthening reactions.
    - By obtaining a contraction of agonist group, the antagonist group relaxes.
    - A series of contraction of antagonists (tight) group caused by therapist applying quick and control stretch will result in relaxation or lengthening of muscle.

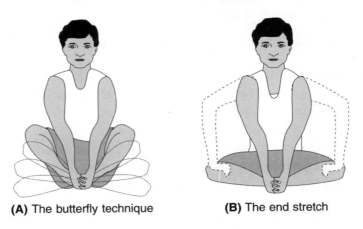

(A) The butterfly technique   **(B)** The end stretch

Figs 13.4A and B: The butterfly and stretch stimulus

When the patient cannot move voluntarily, a series of stretch reflexes, each followed by a responsive muscle contraction and movement may be used resulting in a series of contractions. This aids movement.

"Yogic Sukshmaskriya" of individual joints, can be used as 'repeated contractions' technique, when the extra stretch is the end range gives added rhythm to the movement."

6. *Rhythmic Stabilization:*
   • It is based on isometric muscle work, where there is a simultaneous contraction of all muscles controlling the joint.
   • It can be used to get relaxation or increase muscular strength.

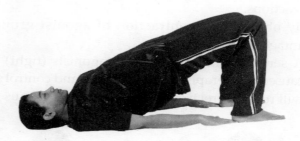

Fig. 13.5: Setubandhasana—Bridging for rhythemic stabilization

7. *Proprioceptive Neuromuscular Facilitation Technique:*
   • Proprioception is essential for movement and learning.
   • Muscle and joint sense is definitely the primary essential requisite for motor control.
   • All the various organs with this type of sensitivity are termed in physiology as the proprioceptive system.
   • *Proprioceptive sense means "sensing itself", i.e. having sense of one's own body.*
   • The kinesthetic system is unique among the sensory systems, in the sense that it is only one that relates directly to the reality.
   • The important factors to be considered in this are Traction, Prolonged stretch, Approximation, Mass movement pattern, Diagonal limb patterns.

The dynamic state of going into and release from an Asana are mass movement patterns, emphasing on the proximal key points of control which also includes in each, a rotatory component at the proximal joint spine, shoulder or hip.

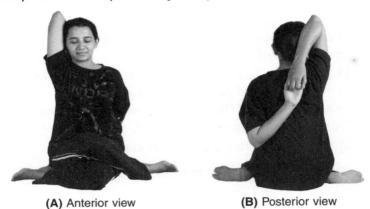

(A) Anterior view   **(B)** Posterior view

Figs 13.6A and B: Gaumukhasana—PNF pattern

- The "commands" are given by "the Self" which facilitate concentration and thereby Stabilization as proprioceptive stimulation enhance summated movements at a will and volition.

The Close kinematic chain pattern of movements resembling the Asanas facilitates 'Approximation' at proximal joints. "The Diagonal Rotatory component is inclusive in all the Yogic postures facilitating proprioception Functional Rehabilitation."

8. *The Reconditioning response:*
    - "A conditioned mind is adjusted and adapted in behaviour."
    - "A conditioned body has flexible joints and relaxed muscles."
    - *A low intensity, repetitive total body movements enhances the three elements of muscle performances.* The Strength, the Power and the Endurance.

- It is related to the body's ability to use oxygen effectively.
- It facilitates response by good oxygen uptake.

The Yogic Breathing technique–Pranayama: Ujjayi is one of the role example for this response.
- It helps Mental and Physical conditioning.
- It strengthens Faith.
- It trains mind to accept difficulties and challenges.
- It makes mind and body free of tension.
- It helps one to be flexible in thoughts and actions.
- This eventually improves day to day performances.
- It strengthens morale and builds confidence.

Table 13.2: Yogic practice and Principles of Exercise therapy

- Hooke's Law.
- Stress-Strain Response.
- Relaxation.
- Stretch Reflex Phenomenon.
- Rhythmic Stabilization.
- Proprioceptive Neuromuscular Facilitation.
- The Reconditioning Response.
- Principles of Mobility.
- Principles of Strengthening.
- Functional Re-education.

THE FUNDAMENTAL STARTING POSTURES\ IN EXERCISE THERAPY AND YOGA

Table 13.3: The fundamental starting of positions Yoga and exercise therapy

Starting position	Asana	Meaning	Benefit
Standing:	Tadasana	(The Tree Pose)	Firmness
Sitting:	Dandasana	(The Long Sitting)	Stability
Supine lying:	Shavasana	(The Corpse Pose)	Relaxation
Prone lying:	Makarasana	(The Crocodile Pose)	Energy Conservation
Side lying:	Dhradasana	(The Balanced Pose)	Digestion

1. Fundamental Standing Position: Tadasana

- We spend hours standing, but never realize or never give a thought as to whether we stand correctly.
- A wrong standing posture leads to uneven pressures on the cartilage of joints of lower limbs and back.
- The basic standing posture helps us to teach correct standing thereby with its regular practise improves standing position.
- Regular practise of this Asana regulates the breath, controls the body, gives stability and firmness.
- It inculcates a feeling of determination, dedication and sound decision-making.
- It is foundation of an "Erect Posture Concept Application."

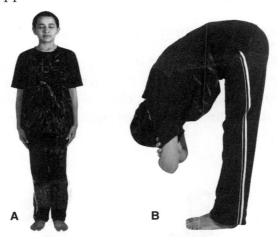

Figs 13.7A and B: (A) Fundamental standing position—Tadasana **(B)** Derived standing position—Uttanasana

Therapeutic Benefits: Uttanasana (Fig. 13.7B)

- *Strengthens all antigravity muscles through Postural mechanism facilitation (Eccentric contraction in close kinematic chain pattern)*

- *Stretches* all posterior muscles – *Tendo achillis, Hamstrings, Back extensors and Thoraco-dorsal fascia.*
- **"One** of the best A**sana to prevent and correct postural problems."**
- **Improves** Respiratory functions.
- Chest is expanded and breath/air exhaled gradually as one lowers down.
- **Improves** endurance through Relaxation. "Concentration throughout the process with breath regulation causes reciprocal relaxation of muscles after release of the Asana."
- **Principle of reactive hyperaemia:** Improves vascularity in all tissues and organs, thereby improves tissue health and vitality.
- A relaxing posture for heart ailments also.

2. Fundamental Sitting Posture: Dandasana

- 'Danda' means stick or rod.
- Most of the time we are sitting in high – sitting posture or supported sitting on a chair, where hips and knees are always in acutely flexed position.

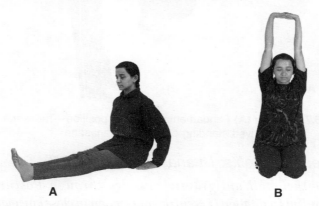

A   B

Figs 13.8A and B: (A) Fundamental sitting position—Dandasana
(B) Derived sitting position—Veerasana

- A wrong sitting position puts uneven weight bearing load on both the ischeal tuberosities causing asymmetrical soft tissue pathologies.
- This posture maintains the physiological length of Hamstrings, facilitating normal lumber lordosis.
- Breathing is also facilitated due to significant expansion of chest in vertical dimension. It is foundation of all other sitting Asana to be practised.

Therapeutic Effects of Veerasana (Fig. 13.8 B)

- It is one of the best **recovery poses** from any illness.
- It gives good rest to the legs.
- If one has stood for long time, walked, cycled or played games or worked, it **recharges the legs** for second round of exercises if required – very beneficial pose for sports personals.
- **All lower limb problems can be prevented due to their "realignment"**.
- If one has lower limb problems, then this Asana should be done with modifications. It will not only relieve pain but prevent further deterioration.
- **Prevents Respiratory dysfunctions** and a useful posture for relaxation for asthmatics.
- "A great relaxing and relieving posture for neck and back problems."
- A Relaxing posture for all **women's issues** like menstrual pain, Antenatal care, etc.

3. Supine Lying Posture: Shavasana (Lying on Back)

- Initially it was believed that this posture (Shavasana) could be practised only in lying, but recently concept has changed. You can do this Asana in any position, time and place. **But Yoga believes it to be practised in lying position.**

- "It is one of the best 'Relaxation' position."
- It should be practised regularly and can be practised by any age group.

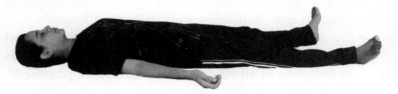

Fig. 13.9: The fundamental supine lying pose—Shavasana

- "It is compared with the Jacobson's Progressive Muscular Relaxation Technique. (JPMR)."
- There are three main steps for muscular relaxation in Shavasana:
  - Be aware of the body parts from distal to proximal, i.e. toes to head.
  - If any discomfort in any part, notice it, feel it closely and then re-arrange the part.
  - Relaxation.
- Throughout the session keep the eyes closed.

Therapeutic Effects of Shavasana (Fig. 13.9)

- Its main effect is to reduces mental stress hence facilitates relief from migraine, blood pressure disturbances, asthma, gastric, and intestinal ulcers, etc.
- Research has proved its effect on Coronary Artery diseases, Auto-immune disorders, Skin problems, Obesity and many psychosomatic disorders.
- A pain relieving posture in painful syndromes.
- It improves concentration and meditative states of mind, which helps one to re-program the mind. It improves stress coping mechanism.
- Through this re-programming it helps to to cope with maladaptive behaviour problems.

- It also improves endocrine and autonomic nervous system functioning, thereby achieving a state of homeostasis.
- General metabolism improves.

4. Prone Lying (Lying on Abdomen): Makarasana

- It is also a "relaxation" posture but practised in prone lying (lying on belly).
- The distance between two legs can be 1 to 2 feet, with toes pointing out.
- Palms clasped and placed under forehead.
- Face could be either to right, left or in centre.
- Free, regulated breath watching.

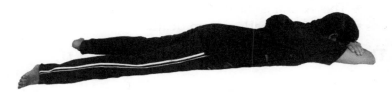

Fig. 13.10: The prone lying pose—Makarasana—The Crocodile Pose

- This Asana is practised in between two Asanas of prone lying, to take rest.

Therapeutic Effects of Makarasana (Fig. 13.10)

- All benefits of Shavasana
- Helps in reducing abdominal fats to some extent.
- Inspite of such heavy weight, a crocodile can move swiftly. It has very little food intake. After heavy activity it again assumes a relaxed steady pose and **Conserves energy**.
- Morale to be followed from the crocodile is to conserve energy through mind regulation and control.

5. Side-Lying Position: Dhradasana

- It is also one of the relaxing position especially after meals.
- It is also having a moral value.
- After meals to lie down in this position to the right side for at least ten to fifteen minutes and then turn to left side.
- *The Moral:* Man is constantly running after material gains and thus lives in stress. There is no scope for rest. Even food, which is said to be fuel supply to body, is consumed in haste. This invites misery and ill health, giving fatal outcome eventually. Hence respecting the food intake, one should rest for sometime with a feeling of gratification.
- This Asana is the only Asana practised after meals.
- Makes one fearless from death.

Therapeutic Effects of Dhradasana (Fig. 13.11)

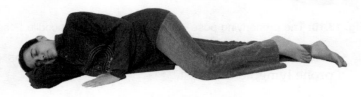

Fig. 13.11: The side lying pose—Dhradasana

- A very positive result for patients of Heart Ailments and Coronary Artery Diseases.
- A relaxing pose during and after asthma attack.
- Prevents all digestion irregularities and facilitates good function of absorption of nutrients and elimination of wastes from body.
- A recommended posture for Hemiplegics and Hemiparatics to prevent and overcome **Abnormal Reflex Tonal Postures and Activity**.

SUMMARY

1. If all these five postures are practised regularly, sincerely and psychophysically, one can lead a life filled with calmness, contentment and complete health.
2. All these posture have no contraindications or side effects and can be practised by all, irrespective of time, place and position.
3. Who can understand better about these poses better than a physiotherapist with the knowledge of biomechanics and exercise therapy.

Chapter 14

YOGA AND REHABILITATION IN RESPIRATORY CONDITIONS

"It is noteworthy that those living creatures who breathe more slowly tend to live longer than those with rapid breathing rates."

— Longitivity of Life.

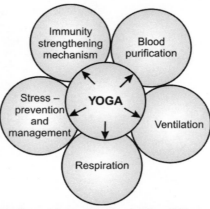

Fig. 14.1: Yoga and its application in Respiratory conditions

THE BREATH OF LIFE

- Many physiological processes are essential to human life. But one physiological function seems to us most important and intimately connected with life is **breathing**. We can survive without food for weeks, without water for days, but without air, our survival has to be measured in seconds.

Hence, it becomes very essential for all of us living in this world to understand the value of this vital source of energy-

"Our Breath"

Know Breath Know Life-Sri Sri Ravishankar,
Breath is said to be charioteer of life.
Breath is the governing force of our life.

- *It is law of nature that as the mind is distracted and diverged. So, is the breath and respiration rapid and irregular.* The activities of both the mind and breath are interconnected.
- More important than physical cleansing is cleansing of mind of its disturbing emotions like hatred, passion, anger, lust, greed, delusion and pride. Such emotions through autonomic nervous system cause bronchospasm affecting the breathing mechanism.
- Our Physical health, growth and purification of blood and consequently the activities of internal organs depend entirely upon the respiratory process.

THE RESPIRATORY SYSTEM

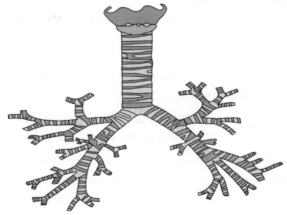

Fig. 14.2A: Upper respiratory tract
Breathing exercises has maximum effect on these segment Puraka-inhalation and Rechaka-Exhalation facilitates cleansing of channels

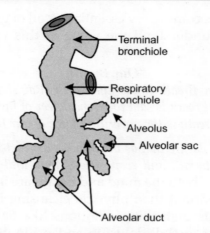

Terminal bronchiole

Respiratory bronchiole

Alveolus

Alveolar sac

Alveolar duct

Fig. 14.2B: Bronchopulmonary segment
Pranayama Kumbhaka (Breath Hold) has maximum effect on this segment and facilitates gas exchange

Physiology of Respiration

It consists of:
1. Ventilation: Inhalation and Exhalation.
2. Gaseous Exchange.
3. Carriage of oxygen and carbondioxide by blood.

1. Ventilation

- Mass exchange of the air into and from the body during inspiration and expiration.
- Movements of the chestwall, inflation and deflation of lungs, flow of air into or out from the lungs.
- **Breathing exercises improve ventilatory functions.**
- The efficacy of gas exchange and adequacy of internal respiration depends on sound and clear ventilatory passage.

2. Gas Exchange

- *Respiration:* It is the general term used to describe gas exchange within body.
- It comprises of:
  - *External Respiration:* Gas exchange between alveolar capillary bed and pulmonary capillaries.
  - *Internal Respiration:* Gas exchange between pulmonary capillaries and cells of the surrounding tissues.
- Deep breathing exercise improve gaseous exchange.
- Pranayama has main effect on Respiratory function.
- The efficacy of tissue health, body health and vitality depends on good respiratory function.

3. Carriage of Oxygen and Carbondioxide by Blood

Cardio-vascular system and cardiorespiratory system are inherently linked. Oxygen passes through the alveoli to the blood vessels, which is then carried to heart to circulate in the body and carbon dioxide passes from blood vessels to the alveoli which expirate it out.

- **Concentration** and **Meditation** have main effect on this function *(Dharna and Dhyana)*
- The sense of well-being in all situations depends make on this aspect.

THE THORACIC CAGE: THE CHEST WALL

- It is made up of sternum (chest bone) anteriorly, 12 thoracic vertebrae posteriorly and the ribs that connects these two structures.
- There are multiple axial and non-axial gliding joints between these bones that facilitate chest expansion in all three directions.

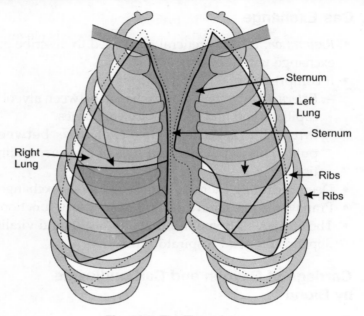

Fig. 14.3: The Thoracic cage

Functions of Thoracic Cage

- **Protects** organs of respiration, circulation and digestion.
- **Participates** in ventilation by its amazing dynamic components of movements.
- **Provides** attachment to muscles of respiration.
- **Provides** attachment to muscles of upper extremity to facilitate breathing.

Movements of Thoracic Cage

It moves in three directions during inspiration:

1. *Vertical dimension:* **The Piston action.** The central tendon of the Diaphragm can descend downwards to about 8 to 10 centimetres with full inspiration. This facilitates effective elevation of ribs which in result enhances vertical expansion of lungs too.

2. *Transverse dimension:* **The Bucket handle action.** This is also called as lateral costal expansion. There is elevation and outward turning of lateral portion of ribs.
3. *Anteroposterior dimension:* **The Pump handle action.** The forward-backward expansion is favored by erect posture. There is forward upward movement of sternum and the upper ribs.

"Erect posture, relaxed mind, flexible joints of shoulder girdle and good strength of muscles controlling it, maintains sound functions of thoracic cage mechanism in all three directions."

MECHANISM OF VENTILATION

1. *Inspiration:* – Contraction of the muscles-diaphragm and intercostal.
   – Expansion of the chest wall.
   – Expansion of the lungs.
   – Sub atmospheric pressure changes in the respiratory tract.
   – Air enters in the respiratory passage.

Good functional inhalation gains energy, vitality and vigour in the body.

2. *Expiration:* – Contraction ceases on its own, approximately after two seconds.
   – Lungs retract because of elastic recoil.
   – Excess atmospheric pressure.
   – Air moves out.
   – It is a passive phenomenon.

It gains calmness, tranquility and relaxation of mind.

Muscles of Ventilation

Lungs are not muscular but they have elasticity, hence good lung volumes and capacities depend on muscles of respiration.

Muscles of Inspiration

- *Diaphragm:* – It is a dome shaped muscle at rest and is a major muscle of inspiration.
  - It flattens and descends down when it contracts.
  - In normal breathing, the downward excursion is about 1.5 to 2 cm.
  - In deep breathing, the downward excursion can be 8 to 10 cm.
  - It is mainly responsible for increasing vertical dimension of chest wall.
  - Performs 70 to 80% of breathing.
  - It is fairly resistant to fatigue. It is an important muscle for Yogic breath.
- *Intercostals:* – External intercostals facilitate rib movements and opening of ribs.
  - Increases transverse diameter and aids antero-posterior dimension of thoracic cage.
- *Scalenii:* – Responsible for pump handle mechanism of rib cage.
  - Work as stabilizers to favour upper rib elevation and expansion.
  - Facilitate upper and outward action of rib cage.
- *Accessory:* – In normal breathing they are not in action.
  Muscles – Active, during deep and labored inspiration.
  - When diaphragm activity reduces, laborious breathing is performed by them.

Muscles of Expiration

- In quiet breathing expiration is a passive process so no muscle actively responsible.

- In forced breathing:
  (i) *Abdominals*: – Good tone of abdominals facilitate diaphragm action.
    – Help to force down thoracic cage and force the abdominal viscera superiorly to push air out of lungs.
  (ii) *Pectoralis major*:
    – Its stabilising action helps in depression of the rib cage.
    – This close kinematic chain work, fixes the arm and promotes chin up and down movements or forward backward movements and aids expiration.

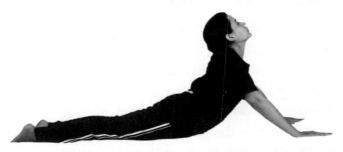

Fig. 14.4: Sarpasana—The snake pose and expiration

PRESSURE CHANGES

1. *In Inspiration:*

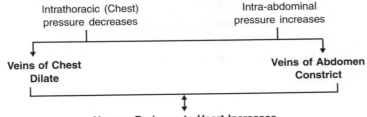

2. *In Expiration:*

- The reverse occurs in expiration.
- These changes are exaggerated in exercises as breathing is uncontrolled whereas in Yogic breathing it is not, as the breathing is controlled.

"In Pranayama, the vertical dimension of the thoracic expansion is facilitated specially in Anulom-vilom (alternate nostril breathing) and Ujjayi (the victorious breath), which leads to all alveoli opening up and out evenly. This leads to controlled pressure changes on expiration facilitating gas exchange at alveolar capillary bed."

ALVEOLAR VENTILATION

- It is the amount of air utilised for gas exchange.
- The alveolar ventilation-perfusion ratio governs the amount of blood that perfuses the alveoli.
- Normally according to posture of body, there is mismatch between ventilation and perfusion.
- In erect posture the ventilation at apices of lungs is good but because of gravity, perfusion is poor, so gaseous exchange does not occur effectively.
- During exercise, the blood supply to apices is also good as blood vessels dilate, so gas exchange is very effective.

"Pranayama, the regulation of voluntary breath technique has maximum effect on ventilation-perfusion ratio as the mind is relaxed, posture is also relaxed and the breathing cycle is continuously regulated. So as long is the kumbhaka, better will be the perfusion. Hence, Pranayama is called as "Soul of Yogic science.""

Regulation of Ventilation: The Rajyoga Effects

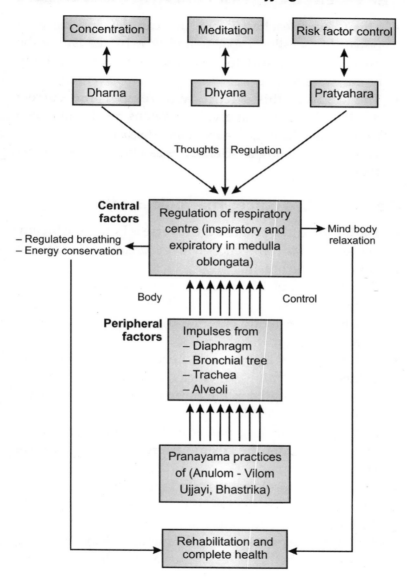

Fig. 14.5: Yogic practice, Respiration and Complete Health

THE SCIENCE OF YOGIC BREATH: PRANAYAMA

- This science teaches us how we can develop the lung power to its fullest capacity and how by regulating the breath, we can purify the cells, tissues and organ activity of our system.
- The study of this science with regular and correct breathing exercise can give marvellous results and keep us in perfect health, free from any disease.
- To know more on this science it is essential to know what **Prana** is.

Prana: The Life Force: The Yogic Breath

- The life force that moves the Universe is Prana, the Breath.
- Our earthly life commences with the breath and ends with passing of the breath.
- If there is enough life force, the organs will destroy all the germs of the disease and also all the microbes and bacteria which are constantly entering into our bodies through breath, food and water.
- Abundance of life force is necessary to resist their influence or to drive them away, or to destroy them and eventually bring back the normal condition which we understand as **Health**.
- **In Yoga this healing power of life force is called the Prana. Breathing the cosmic energy can help achieve Prana**.
- The perfect control over the mind and body can be reached by controlling the motion of the lungs. And controlling the motion of the lungs is Pranayama.
- Pranayama helps in silencing the mind, thereby regulating the rate and rhythm of respiration and facilitating Energy conservation.

- Pranayama, the Yogic breathing exercise cleanses the intellect of impure thoughts and facilitates ventilation and respiration through Autonomic nervous system.

"Most of the respiratory diseases are the result of poor immune system. Healing the mind, heals the body by strengthening of the immune system."

"A healthy and sound respiratory system is a result of powerful life force within."

"Healthy respiratory system nurtures well, all other systems hence breath is life."

THE VALUE OF CORRECT BREATHING

- Correct breathing improves the immune system and protects one from all diseases.
- *Nostril breathing:* Breathing should always be practised through nose.
- The oxygen of the air entering through the open door of the lungs filter through the thin walls of pulmonary capillaries, comes in contact with venous blood, produces a kind of combustion and destroys all the impure matter that is deposited in the blood and as a result of combustion, carbonic acid gas is generated which comes out in form of impure breath.
- Ordinarily, we use only one sixth of full lung capacity. If we use the whole capacity for daily use, the results would be encouraging. This is the benefit of correct breathing.
- *The Yogic breathing:*
  - **Develops** power of the lungs.
  - **Uses** fullest capacities of the lungs.
  - **Draws** largest quantity of oxygen from the atmosphere.
  - **Regulates** the whole respiratory process and the system.

- It is the key for attaining the desirable physiological and psychological harmony
- **Helps** to reduce oxygen debt and increase oxygen reservoir.
- **Reduces** respiratory rate and prevents exhaustion—mental and physical.
- **Conserves** energy of all types and of all systems.
- **Prevents** obstructive lung disorders and helps in reversing their symptoms.
- **Should be regularly practised by one and all for Complete health and Rehabilitation in all dimensions of life.**

Role of Diaphragm in Yogic Breathing

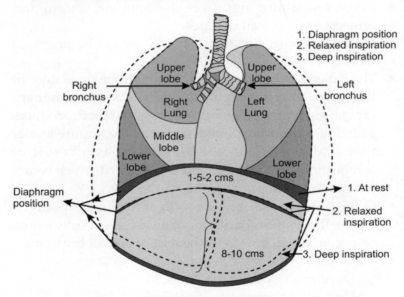

Fig. 14.6: Pranayama and diaphragmatic breathing

• The normal sequence of inspiration by diaphragm is usually as follows:

- The diaphragm contracts and descends and the epigastric area of the abdomen rises.
- The vertical excursion gives firm anchorage to the two lateral ends of diaphragm in Padmasana (the lotus posture), facilitating lateral costal expansion
- This then raises the upper chest effectively.
- The contraction and relaxation of diaphragm with its 8-10 cm excursion gives micromassage effect to heart and lungs upwards and to liver, spleen, pancreas and other abdominal and pelvic organs downwards.
- This improves overall physiological functioning of the body
- Moreover the improved ventilation also aids expiration by diaphragmatic relaxation.
- By gradually slowing down the respiratory rate and rhythm, prolonging the inhalation and exhalation more and more and leaving as long an interval as possible between these two movements helps reduce the rate of respiration and enhances conservation of energy.
- Diaphragmatic breathing thus promotes mental and physical relaxation.

"If the Prana is unevenly controlled, the whole nervous system will be agitated and the results will be dangerous. Controlling the breath gradually first by thoughts regulation, will power strengthening and then controlling over the activities of lungs through diaphragm, prevents and overcomes many respiratory problems."

THE INTEGRATED APPROACH

The Physiotherapy Assessment

1. *The Posture:* Hyperextended head position obliterates free expiration.

2. The thoracic and shoulder girdle mobility.

3. The thoracic and shoulder girdle muscle dynamics.

4. The breathing patterns.

5. Type of breathing pattern, where the patient breathes, upper or lower parts of lungs.

6. Respiratory rate and rhythm.

7. Special signs as per the respiratory disorder.

8. The Personality traits (Psychosomatic cause).

9. The Environmental factors.

10. The person's attitude and inclination towards the whole management programme.

The Goals of the Integrated Approach

1. **Prevent or correct:** postural deformities associated with the respiratory disorders.

2. **Maintain** and improves chest and shoulder girdle mobility (Sukshmakriyas).

3. **Improve** strength and endurance of postural muscles (Asanas, Pranayama).

4. **Conserve** energy through breath retraining and regulation (Pranayama Meditation).

5. **Prevent** accumulations of secretions and airway obstruction that interfere with normal respiration (Yogic cleansing method of bellow breath-Bhastrika and Alternate nostril breathing).

6. **Improve** airway clearence and ventilation.(Pranayama).

7. **Improve** endurence (Pranayama).

8. **Promote** relaxation (Pranayama).

9. **Life style modifications** (Pratyahara, Pranayama and Diet).

THE YOGIC LIFE STYLE FOR ASTHAMATICS

1. **Yama and Niyama:** *"Prevention is better then cure."*
   - Yogic practise has better effect on modifiable functional disorders. Asthama is a reversible disorder hence Asthama is only being mentioned here. Though this can be followed by all.
     a. **Positive health:** The attitude needs to be positive for better results.
     b. **Avoid smoking.**
     c. Avoid **dampness and dust,** both for mind and body.
     d. Avoid **stress** and **anxiety** and hot confrontations whenever and wherever possible.
     e. Avoid jerky quick movements and **impulsive** acts.
     f. Use cotton and synthetic mattresses rather than feather and fur.
     g. Sensible eating habits. Avoid **cold, refrigerated and tinned** food.
     h. Improve communication abilities and skills
     i. Group therapy is very beneficial as one can have positive outlets, *"Satsang."*
     j. Aerobic activity like swimming and cycling can be encouraged
     k. Regularity, sincerity and dedication in Yogic practise, be recommended.
     l. A transparent, flexible, approachable, pleasant personality development.

"Strengthen stress coping mechanism- mental and physical at all levels of functioning."

2. **The Yogasana**
   a. They have great effects on all Restrictive lung disorders as they encourage thoracic expansion.

b. **Mobilize** indirectly all small joints of thoracic cage by gliding of acromio-clavicular, sterno-clavicular and costo-vertebral joints.

c. **Strengthen** the stabilizers of shoulder girdle which aids in chest expansion.

d. **Prevent** and **correct** postural deviations of cervical and lumber lordosis.

e. This **enhance** free diaphragmatic excursion and chest expansion.

f. Improves inspiratory capacity hence is said to be **"Energizing component of body"**

3. **The Yogic Breath: Pranayama**

   Know breath: Know life

   a. It has great effects on Obstructive lung disorders as it **reduces** and **relaxes** bronchospasm, it facilitates diaphragmatic relaxation and aids in regulated rhythmic breathing.

   b. Regulating the breath regulates the mind, **relaxes** the physique, as the breath is the connecting link between mind and body.

   c. It leads to **decreased adreno-cortical activity** therefore increases ability to resist stress.

   d. Use of full lung capacity, therefore cardiac functions also improve due to improved gas exchange thereby increasing physiological resistance too.

   e. **Improves** expiratory capacity hence said to be "Relaxing component of body."

   f. *Ujjayi and Anulom-Vilom* Pranayama are beneficial for these conditions.

4. **Yogic Diet: Pratyahara:** Along with life style modifications, diet regulation also helps in prevention and reversion.

Table 14.1: The Yogic diet in Asthama

Food to avoid	Food recommended
- Sweets and dairy products	- Fresh vegetarian diet.
- Vegetables like pumpkin, cauliflower	- Vegetables green leafy
- Grains like rice and masoor	- Grains like wheat, pulses beans
- Bakery items like bread burgers, pizzas	- Baked, roasted and raw food good
- Stale, refined, preservatives	- Hot, warm, fresh soups and food
- Fried items and refrigerated food items	- Salt very useful if no associated problems
	- Honey

THE THERAPEUTIC EFFECTS OF YOGIC PRACTICE

- This is the thing unknown to the Psychologist and Medical practioners quote the yoga experts.
- Through all kinds of breathing exercises, diseases can be cured, but in yogic breathing, it is not only oxygen intake, but intake of different powers too. This power is not oxygen nor electricity nor molecular attraction, but it is a nervous energy called the life force which strengthens the stress coping mechanisms and improves one's immune system.
- Regulated, controlled and correct breathing gains self control, peace, calmness and tranquility leading to a state of harmony, preventing many Psychosomatic lung disorders like Asthama, Bronchitis, Tuberculosis (A result of poor immunity).
- Senses are drawn inwards. A feeling of "look within" develops. Self analysis and introspection improves acceptance and tolerance levels of an individual thereby accelerating the recovery process from **disabling lung disorders**.

- Pranayama and Meditation aid mental and physical relaxation and hence reduce stress levels of mind and body thus overcoming **Respiratory fatigue syndromes**.
- Yogic postures of all the three types prevent most of the restrictive lung disorders (Relaxation, Meditation, Cultural Asanas).

SUMMARY

1. In respiratory disorders a physiotherapist does not treat a "diagnosis" but uses all techniques available to her, to help solve patient's problems, I feel so.
2. In COPD, medically there is still no agreement on value of breathing exercise as palliative treatment. Focus is on relaxation - The ultimate goal of Yoga is energy conservation through relaxation.
3. Chronic stress triggers, precipitates, and aggravates asthma attacks and episodes by reducing efficacy of the adrenal glands of its anti-inflammatory response. Yogic practise results into a state of homeostasis: physiological balance between ANS and the Endocrine glands.
4. Respiratory disorders are reversible. Understanding the cause is important than treating the symptoms for long lasting effects always.
5. Any technique chosen should not cause bronchospasm.

"By gaining control over life force, we get physical, mental, moral and spiritual results with potential effects on rehabilitation."

L Chapter 15

YOGA AND REHABILITATION IN CARDIOVASCULAR CONDITIONS

"It is more important to know what kind of patient has the disease, then what kind of disease the patient has."

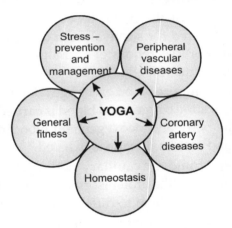

Fig. 15.1: Yoga and cardiovascular conditions

INTRODUCTION

No two illnesses are alike, though the labels are put and attempt made to group them, but *in fact every person is ill in his own way and his way of life depends on what he is, on his state of consciousness and the life he leads.*

Cardiovascular diseases are generally the leading cause of death today. This marked increase is seen primarily in the Western industrialised societies and can be regarded *as manifestations of civilisation and progress.*

These diseases *cause a great economic burden in the patient's family and community* in terms of money spent on health care and loss of income.

To have the cardiovascular system function normally in modern day life, is a great boon.

FUNCTIONS OF CARDIOVASCULAR SYSTEM

1. *Transportation*: It is responsible for transportation of respiratory gases. Inhaled oxygen is transported to different parts of the body. Blood transports different minerals required for survival from one part to another. It also transports secretions of hormones to target organs secreted by endocrine glands.

2. *Respiration:* Impure blood exchange takes place in lungs. After purification oxygenated blood is carried to different cells of the body and deoxygenated blood reaches back to lungs and carbon dioxide is exhaled.

3. *Nutrition:* Abundant capillary bed in small intestine, absorbs nutrients like proteins, glucose and vitamins from food and supplies them to different cells of the body.

4. *Excretion*: The eliminated minerals in form of waste products are excreted through lungs and kidneys (urea, ammonia, creatine, etc.)

5. *Temperature regulation of the body*: Body temperature is evenly maintained with its close functioning with ANS.

6. *Defence function*: Lymphocytes are mainly responsible for immunity and neutrophils are to destroy dead cells.

"This system acts as exchanger, transporter and disassociator."

STRUCTURE OF CARDIOVASCULAR SYSTEM

The main organs to form this system are Heart, Blood vessels (artereries and veins) and Blood.

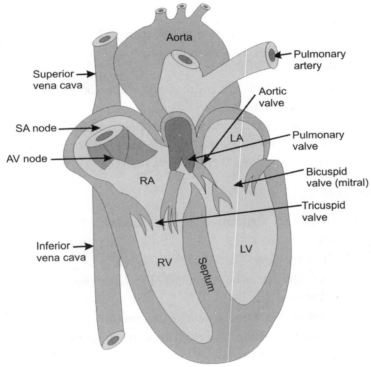

Fig. 15.2: Heart and vessels

Heart

1. It is a fist-sized muscular sac weighing approximately 250-350 gms in a normal adult.
2. It comprises of four chambers: *Upper two atriums* and *lower two ventricles*.
3. All four chambers perform different functions. The two right chambers carry **impure blood** and the two left chambers carry **pure blood**.

4. The *muscles of heart* are smooth muscles and are under the control of ANS.

5. **Valves of the heart:** Main four valves which strictly maintain one way circulation.
   • They do not allow mixture of impure and pure blood.
   • Mitral valve connects left atrium to left ventricle and tricuspid valve connects the right atrium to right ventricle.
   • The other two are pulmonary valve to the lungs and aortic valve to aorta.

6. **Sino-atrial node:** It is known as pacemaker of the heart and it regulates rate and rhythm of the heart. AV node is known as reserve pacemaker of heart.

Vessels

They are tubular structures carrying blood.

1. *Arteries*
   a. They are deep seated and thick walled.
   b. They carry pure oxygenated blood from heart to tissues of the body.
   c. Their appearance is scarlet red colour.
   d. Blood pressure is relatively high in the arteries compared to veins.
   e. Pulmonary artery carries impure blood from right ventricle to lungs and it is the only artery in the body to carry deoxygenated blood.

2. *Veins*
   a. They are superficially located and thin walled.
   b. They carry impure deoxygenated blood from tissues and organs of the body towards heart.
   c. Pulmonary vein carries pure blood from lungs to left atrium and it is the only vein in the body to carry oxygenated blood.

3. *Capillaries*
   a. They are microscopic vessels that connect arterioles and venules.
   b. They have the largest surface area in the body.

Blood

1. It is not a liquid but it is a solid content of the body.
2. It is made up of blood plasma (55%) and cells (45%).
3. It is continuously circulating in the vessels.
4. Its volume is approximately 5 to 6 litres. This volume is limited and it has to perform unlimited functions of the body continuously to meet its demands.
5. This volume is used over and over again. If proper care not taken to maintain its functions then many cardiovascular problems may be invited.

"Yogic practise maintains its resiliency throughout life and prevents any type of cardiovascular problems."

Physiology of Circulation

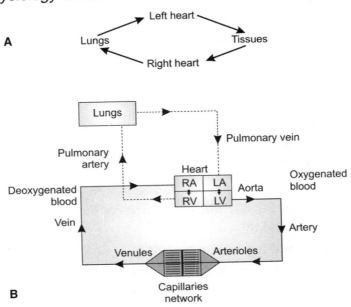

Figs. 15.3A and B: **(A)** Basic circulation **(B)** Physiology of circulation

SOME IMPORTANT ASPECTS TO KNOW FOR YOGIC PRACTISE

1. *Vasodilatation*: It is a state of increase in the diameter of the vessels.

2. *Vasoconstriction*: It is a state of decrease in the diameter of the vessels.

3. *Heart muscles*:

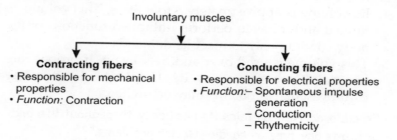

"Yogic practise induces reciprocal relaxation of heart muscles and facilitates conduction."

4. *SA node*: • Pacemaker of the heart.
   • Regulates rate and rhythm of the heart.
   • Connected to the higher centres in brain through autonomic nervous system.

"Yogic practise prevents and reduces overload on SA Node function. Pranayama and Meditation have been proved to cause this effect through relaxation."

5. *Heart rate*:
   • Normal: 75 -80/ minute (In present day life stresses)
   • Controlled by –
   a. Neural mechanism (ANS).
   b. Chemical reactions (Adrenaline, Thyroxin)
   c. Thermal changes (Temperature)

- It is directly proportional to the need of oxygen of the cardiac muscles.
- It increases with emotional stress, exertional exercises diseases and other factors.

"Yogic practise in form of certain cultural asana, and all relaxation and meditative asanas help in maintaining and regulating the normal heart rate in time of crisis. One cannot overlook the importance of meditation in regulating the total system."

6. *Blood pressure*:
   - Normal: 120- 80/mm Hg
   - It is directly proportional to heart rate.
   - It increases with stress, over exertion (mental), certain metabolic disorders, etc.
   - Diastole-filling of the blood in the heart, peripheral circulation is lowered and coronary circulation is increased. **It is a state of relaxation of heart.**
   - Systole-emptying of the blood from the heart, peripheral circulation is increased and coronary circulation is decreased. **It is a state of contraction of the heart.**

"Yogic practise through parasympathetic activity has maximum effect on diastolic blood pressure, aiding relaxation of heart muscles, increasing coronary circulation to meet the demands of aerobic activity of the heart muscles, thereby preventing and reversing the consequences of cardiovascular disorders."

7. *Regulation of the pumping of heart* (contraction and relaxation)

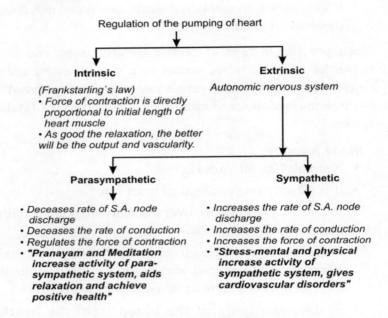

"The purpose of regulating the pumping effect by yogic practice is to strengthen the effectiveness of parasympathetic nervous system and control the overactivity of the sympathetic nervous system."

8. *Regulation of the blood pressure:*

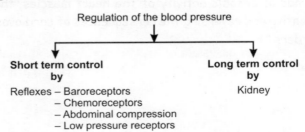

a. ***Baroreceptor reflex:*** It is a very important reflex and is sensitive to rapidly changing pressures and postures.

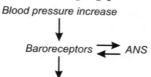

Blood pressure increase

↓

Baroreceptors ⇌ *ANS*

↓

- *Reduces blood pressure*
- *Reduces heart rate*
- *Vasodilatation*
- *Reduced force of contradiction*

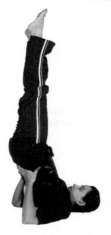   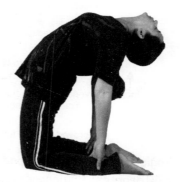

(A) Modified Sarvangasana —Neck flexed   **(B)** Ushtrasana—Neck extended

Figs 15.4A and B: Asanas facilitating baroreceptor activity

"Yogic postures, specifically the inverted postures greatly influence this regulation and control blood pressure."

- But the practise should be started after thorough medical assessment and under proper guidance.
- The postures which positively helps for blood pressure regulation are Shirsasana, (the head stand posture) Sarvangasana, Matsyasana, (fish posture) Ushtrasana (camel posture).
- These Asanas should be practised for prevention programmes.

- These Asanas should not be practised in cervical spondylosis.
- Management programme should be only after professional assessment and under Yogic guidance.

b. *Abdominal compression reflex:*

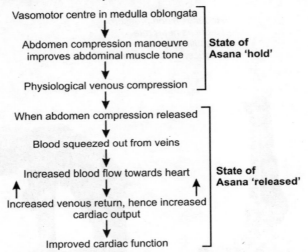

```
Vasomotor centre in medulla oblongata  ┐
              ↓                         │
Abdomen compression manoeuvre           │  State of
improves abdominal muscle tone          │  Asana 'hold'
              ↓                         │
Physiological venous compression       ┘
              ↓
When abdomen compression released      ┐
              ↓                         │
Blood squeezed out from veins           │
              ↓                         │
Increased blood flow towards heart      │  State of
↑             ↓             ↑           │  Asana 'released'
Increased venous return, hence increased│
            cardiac output              │
              ↓                         │
Improved cardiac function              ┘
```

"Yogic postures like Uttanpadasana (bilateral straight leg raise to 40 degrees), Bhujangasana (the cobra posture), Dhanurasana (the bow pose), Shalabhasana (the locust pose) causes reflex abdominal compression, and if these asanas are practised regularly with psychophysical purpose, it gradually helps in regulating blood pressure (These should be started after complete medical examination and under proper supervision)."

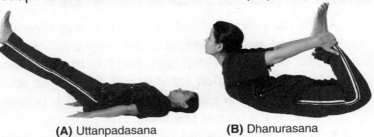

(A) Uttanpadasana   **(B)** Dhanurasana

Figs 15.5A and B: Asanas and abdominal compression reflex

- These Asanas should be practised for prevention programmes.
- These Asanas not to be practised in lumber spondylosis problem.
- There should not be "breath holding" during any stage of Asana.
- Thorough assessment and appropriate Yogic guidance must for management programme.

Cardiac output and Venous return:
- Cardiac output is volume of blood that can be ejected by heart in one minute
- Factors influencing cardiac output are:
  a. Venous return
  b. Force of contraction
  c. Heart rate
  d. Emotions
  e. Muscular exercise
  f. Yogasanas

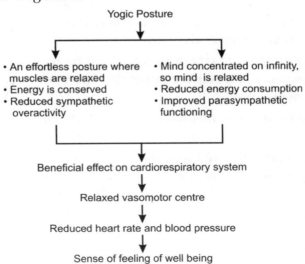

CORONARY ARTERY DISEASE (CAD)

- Certain risk factors are associated with development of this disease. Recent research has clearly established the importance of lifestyle for prevention of heart problems and vascular disorders.
- Cigarette smoking is a risk factor but it is a psycophysiological stressor.
- Along with physical factors psychosocial factors mainly contribute to risk factors for developing coronary artery disorders.
- Let me focus on the risk factors and stressors that cause this problem which is of great concern.

Risk Factors

1. *Lifestyle habits*: Sedentory lifestyle, cigarette smoking, obesity, diet rich in calories, bad cholestrol, saturated fats, increased salt intake etc.
2. *Genetic factors*: Age and sex are predisposing factors.
3. *Unwise* use of drugs, contraceptive pills also have been reported to trigger the cause.
4. *Personality traits* like aggression, hyperactivity, impatience, excessive competitive drive, etc. aggravate the symptoms.
5. *Psychosocial factors* have over-ruled the other causes in present day situations.
6. *Lack of exercise,* reduces exercise tolerance, causing early fatigue and exhaustion.

Table 15.1: Psychopathology and coronary artery disease

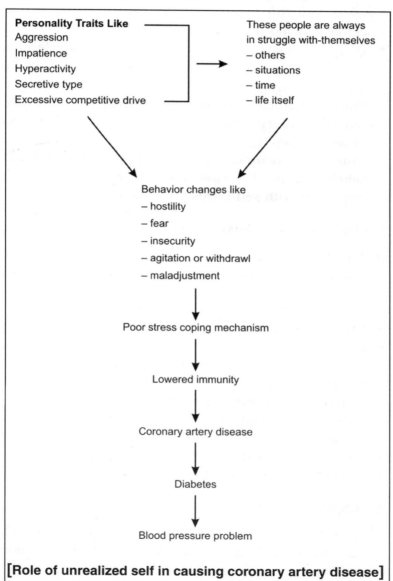

Personality Traits Like
Aggression
Impatience
Hyperactivity
Secretive type
Excessive competitive drive

These people are always
in struggle with-themselves
– others
– situations
– time
– life itself

Behavior changes like
– hostility
– fear
– insecurity
– agitation or withdrawl
– maladjustment

Poor stress coping mechanism

Lowered immunity

Coronary artery disease

Diabetes

Blood pressure problem

[Role of unrealized self in causing coronary artery disease]

The Integrated Approach for Coronary Heart Disease

- Of all the risk factors quoted, 80% of these can be eliminated and reversed.
- With proper and methodical assessment of these factors, Yogic practise and intervention methods, results can be achieved positively and effectively.
- Physical training is not the goal of cardiac rehabilitation. Its prime goal is psychological reassurance and prevention of deconditioning.
- **More than treatment goals and approaches in CAD rehabilitation, it is education and awareness that is important with self-introspection and analysis.**

I. Physiotherapy Assessment

It should be such that it develops and establishes a good, rapport and trust between patient and therapist. It includes assessment of:
- Psychosocial factors.
- Risk factors profile.
- Diet.
- Patient's knowledge of heart disease.
- Personal goals.
- Family environment and relationship.
- Occupational factors, working hours, patterns, pressures, attitude, etc.
- Gross neuromuscular examination.
- Vital organs, chest wall functions.

II. Yogic Practise

- It creates an environment within self and outside which can ensure improved compliance in overall rehabilitation programme.

- It reduces levels of stress anxiety and depression.
- It prevents the consequences of late onset associated problems and recurrence.
- It has revealed significant improvement in cardiovascular system functioning.
- Yogic practise if followed with regularily, sincerely and faith brings equilibrium between the sympathetic and parasympathetic nervous system functioning in 3 to 6 months time thereby balancing the mental and physical functioning too.
- The Ashtangyoga ladder implementation with dedication and determination prevents all adverse consequences in coronary artery functioning and nurtures a healthy heart.

"Yogic lifestyle is safe, economical, drug free, with no side effects, age old authenticity, time tested reliability, prevention oriented with personal meaning and therapy."

III. Yogic Advices: (Yama and Niyama)

- Modify the lifestyle keeping in mind the risk factors.
- Proper, timely sound sleep. "Early to bed and early to rise "concept.
- Relax in "Dhradasana (lying on right side) following afternoon meals for 10 to 15 minutes.
- Control the pace of life by controlling the desires.
- Control the body weight and reduce it if overweight with proper advise and guidance.
- Stop alcohol, smoking and all adverse habits
- Practise good deeds. One good deed a day nourishes the heart and nurtures the soul.

Live with the feeling "I am OK" "You are OK" and "Everything is OK.

- Live in the present and accept life the way it comes.
- Follow the medical and physiotherapy advice with faith and sincerity.
- Aerobic activity for cardiopulmonary endurance in form of walking at least for 30 minutes/day.
- Walking and Asana should be practised with at least 8 hours of interval.

"Self-introspection and self-discipline is a key to prevent and reverse coronary artery diseases."

IV. Yogic Postures: Yogasanas

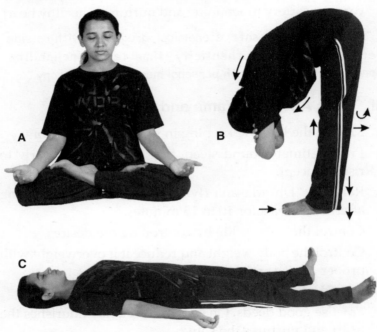

(A) Padamasana **(B)** Uttanasana **(C)** Shavasana

Figs 15.6A to C: Asanas in CAD

These Asana can be safely practised for both, prevention and management programme.

V. Yogic Breathing: Pranayama

- The Yogic cleansing process of Kapalbhati.
- Anulom vilom breathing without retention: Alternate nostril breathing.
- Ujjayi breathing: The victorious breathing.
- In acute care, both above breathing methods can be done in lying.
- In recovering and recovered state, it should be practised in sitting.

VI. Yogic Concentration: Dharana

- Sit in any comfortable posture, preferably meditative posture.
- Visualise the "Anahat chakra" (chest region)
- Auto suggestions   "I am part of Cosmic air."
                      "I am flowing freely like air."
                      "I am here to spread message of love and happiness."
                      "I am full of life."

Time: No time limit, one should practise as per one's capacity.

"Concentration opens the door towards meditation."

VII. Stress Relaxation and Meditation for CAD Patients

- Like the stress response, the relaxation response is also implemented in its own specific part of hypothalamus. Together these two response centres act as antagonists-agonist to control the level of stress activation of the stress response centre.
- This relaxation response acts generally to reduce sympathetic and increase parasympathetic activity. **This is the effect of Meditation on ANS**.

- The more tranquil and focused a person is, the more he is likely to attain a calmer state of bodily function.
- The balance between the sympathetic (energy channelisation) and parasympathetic (energy conservation), facilitates balance between the internal organs.
- Meditation at the scientific end resembles a technique for achieving systemic relaxation, aiding coronary artery function.
- Meditation may lead to an enhanced self-concept which in turn can modify the level at which "eu-stress" (eu means well) exists.

"Meditation has been rediscovered in health care as disease reversal phenomenon".

Some Simple Meditation Techniques for CAD Patient

In any comfortable Yogic posture: Padmasana, Shavasana or Sukhasana.

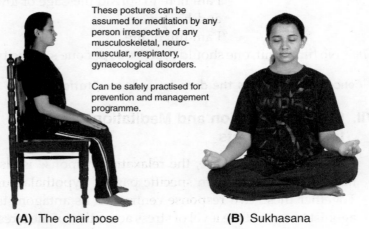

These postures can be assumed for meditation by any person irrespective of any musculoskeletal, neuro-muscular, respiratory, gynaecological disorders.

Can be safely practised for prevention and management programme.

(A) The chair pose   **(B)** Sukhasana

Fig. 15.7: Meditation pose in CAD

(a) *Mantra Dhyana*: (Enchanting silently any mantra of one's faith).

- Aum, Soham, Gayatri Mantra.
- Eyes closed, regulate the mantra with breath control.
- 10 to 15 minutes to begin with, time duration as per capacity.

(b) *Shvasana Dhyana:* (Breath watching meditation)

- Any comfortable Yogic posture, preferably meditative posture.
- Eyes closed and be aware of your breath, concentrate on its rate and rhythm.
- Just be an observer, do not make any effort.
- Time duration to begin with can be by 10-15 minutes.

(c) *Maun Dhyana:* (Silent meditation)

- Any comfortable Yogic posture, preferably meditative posture.
- Eyes closed and divert your thoughts within. Be a passive observer of your thought process.
- Just let the thought pass by silently. Do not resist, neither concentrate nor acknowledge. Just observe.
- This practise should be inculcated in all activities of daily living, at work place, home, walking, etc.

"Silencing the mind is meditation."

Yogic Dietary Advice for CAD

- The nutritional value of the food is of course to be considered always because eating whole and unprocessed food combined with the principles of cooking and eating constitute a **wholistic nutrition.**
- Modifying the food intake according to suggestions of religious belief, temperament, ecological placement, moral and personal satisfaction as its main aim is to tranquilise the mind. Too many constraints frustrate a person.
- Yoga is not possible for him who eats too much nor for him who does not eat at all (fasting as penance). Both these extremes are symptomatic of identifying the body with sensation, as stated in Bhagwad Gita (Pleasure and pain).

- Too much is said, quoted and written about the type of food to be taken by the persons of *CAD by different professionals.*

"The act of eating should be practised as a sacred act with the feeling of dedication, sacrifice, and contentment. This tranquilise the mind, relaxes the body and takes care of all the systems of the body "

PERIPHERAL VASCULAR DISORDERS (PVD)

- Vascular disorders which cause insufficient circulation to the extremities can result in significant physical impairments. These vascular disorders are broadly classified as Acute or Chronic Peripheral Vascular Disease (PVD).
- These disorders may be arterial disorders or venous disorders.
- **Yogic approaches can be beneficial largely to the Chronic, modifiable vascular disorders.**

I. Chronic Vascular Arterial Disorders

- Usually affects lower extremities and is common in elderly patients associated with risk factors that include elevated serum cholesterol, smoking, high blood pressure, obesity and diabetes mellitus.
- Common clinical manifestations are decreased skin temperature, sensory disturbances like tingling, exercise pain and rest pain too in calf muscles and muscles' weakness.

The Integrated Approach

a. **Physiotherapy Assessment and Guidelines:**
   - The physiotherapist has sound understanding of the underlying pathologies and clinical manifestations of many types of arterial, venous, and lymphatic obstructions.

- The physiotherapist is also aware of use, effectiveness, and limitations of therapeutic exercise so that she can be a better guide in rehabilitation of the patients with the Yogic approaches.

b. **Goals of Treatment**
- Decrease ischaemia by restoration and improvement of blood flow.
- Lifestyle modifications and dietary advice like avoid salt and sucrose and fried food.
- Physical therapy may not have much curative effect in these disorders but will minimise the risk factors quotes the litreature.
- **Yogic practise has beneficial effects on these disorders.**

How Yogic Practise Helps?

a. *Yogic Postures:*

Table 15.2: How yogic practice helps in CAD

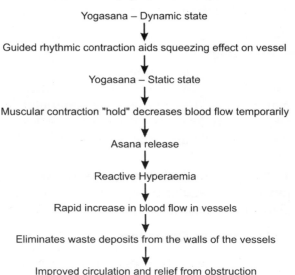

Yogasana – Dynamic state

↓

Guided rhythmic contraction aids squeezing effect on vessel

↓

Yogasana – Static state

↓

Muscular contraction "hold" decreases blood flow temporarily

↓

Asana release

↓

Reactive Hyperaemia

↓

Rapid increase in blood flow in vessels

↓

Eliminates waste deposits from the walls of the vessels

↓

Improved circulation and relief from obstruction

The Asana beneficial are Vajrasana, Padmasana, Uttanpadasana, Pawanmuktasana, Utkatasana.

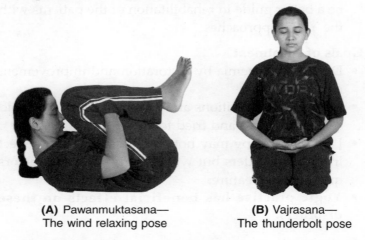

(A) Pawanmuktasana—
The wind relaxing pose

(B) Vajrasana—
The thunderbolt pose

Figs 15.8A and B: Asana in Chronic vascular arterial disorders

"Asanas are psychophysical postures. Regulating the thoughts in the state of Asana tranquilises the mind, improves ANS activity which further aids vasodilation, improving vascularity."

b. *Yogic Breathing:*
   Pranayama: This improves gas exchange at peripheral and central level thereby aiding vascular sufficiency by its cleansing effect. The Pranayama beneficial would be Suryabhedan (right nostril breathing) and Kapalbhati.
c. *The Yogic* lifestyle and diet accelerates the recovering process.
d. *The Yogic* warm ups **Sukshmakriyas of lower limbs**. This is equivalent to regular brisk walking programme daily for 15 to 20 minutes.

II. Chronic Venous Disorders

* Inadequate venous return over a prolonged period of time. Its causes may be varied.

- Chronic pooling of blood in the veins causes inadequate oxygenation of cells and removal of waste products which can lead to venous stasis.
- Dependent peripheral oedema, occurring with long periods of standing or sitting is its common symptom. Oedema decreases as limb is elevated.

The Integrated Approach

- More than the exercise used it is the patient education programme that is important.
- The patient should be given positional advice and educated about self-management.
- Yogasanas and Pranayama are self prescription and self-management skills which take care of both the aspects—the mind and the body.
    a. *Yogic posture:* Shalabhasana, Uttanpadasana, Sarvangasana.

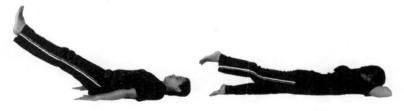

(A) Uttanpadasana   **(B)** Modified
(Bilateral SLR 45°)   Ardhashalabhasana

Figs 15.9A and B: Asana in chronic venous disorders

    b. *Yogic breathing:* Anulom vilom breathing and Bhastrika.
    c. *Yogic lifestyle:* It takes care of the risk factors associated with DVT, obesity and dietary habits.

"Prevention is better than cure in peripheral vascular disorders."

SUMMARY

1 Ninety five percent risk factors listed by WHO are psychosocial stressors.

2. The therapeutic value of Yogic practise in prevention and elimination is more felt then expressed in management in CAD.

3. The integrated approach focuses on muscular relaxation, autogenic training and biofeedback.

4. The tranquilizing effect to control heart rate and BP is achieved by regulating the midbrain reticular action.

5. The sedative effect on mind and body is confirmed by rise in alpha activity as reported by many EEG studies.

"All confirmatively assure and encourage the role of Yogic practise in cardiovascular rehabilitation."

"Where there is will, there is a way."

— A Quotable Quote.

Chapter 16

YOGA AND REHABILITATION IN NEUROMUSCULAR CONDITIONS

"Nervous system is concerned with Physical (Motor, Sensory, Autonomic), Intellectual and Emotional activities, and in consequences, any disorders of Nervous system may involve anyone directly and/or all three of their major functions."

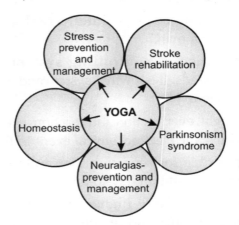

Fig. 16.1: Yoga and its applications in neuromuscular conditions

- Immediately, following any neurological insult which would lead to sudden disablement of a person, to move the body or body parts affected, the individual's response will be primarily at the psychological level. Thus the person goes into the state of psychological shock.

- It is during this phase, if the person is soothed, calmed down, comforted and relaxed emotionally and mentally, the psychological and physical adjustment will be maximum.
- Yogic approach of therapy of Pranayama, Dharna and Dhyana makes the person accept the stress reaction positively and helps him to participate in the rehabilitation process effectively. **Yogic postures aid to the rehabilitation programme** in neuromuscular conditions too.

FUNCTION OF NERVOUS SYSTEM

- It is a very complex system, still not fully understood. Research is still going on extensively to know its hidden capacities and capabilities.
- It is responsible both for **intellectual** and **physical** capabilities of a man.
- It is also called as **controlling system** along with endocrines glands. It is a wired system and endocrine is a wireless system.
- Every thought, every action and reaction, every sensation begins with some electrochemical event in the brain.
- It is responsible for sensation, perception, movement synchronization and all day-to-day activities of life.
- It is also the centre of higher functions of thinking, intelligence, memory and reasoning.
- It is the centre of most important function of emotions and feelings which guides, control, modify and are , applied to the function of a social human being.

BASIC STRUCTURE: NEURON

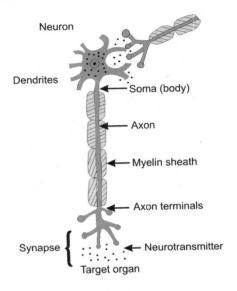

Fig: 16.2: The neuron

- It is believed that about 1.5 crore sensory neurons receive and carry information from the external and internal environment to the central nervous system and about 20 times more than these are involved in transformation of this input impulses through analysis, synthesis, co-ordination, integration and interpretation.

"Yoga science states that there are about 20 times more neurons-nerve cells connected to Gyanendriyas (sense organs) than are those with Karmendriyas (the action organs). Hence, it is so important to regulate, control and balance our sense organs functioning for a stable, balanced disease-free life. It elaborates on Pratyahaar- sense withdrawl from distracting stimuli. The main sutra or aphorism of Sage Patanjali is **"Yoga chitta vritti nirodh."**

CLASSIFICATION OF NERVOUS SYSTEM

As per its Parts

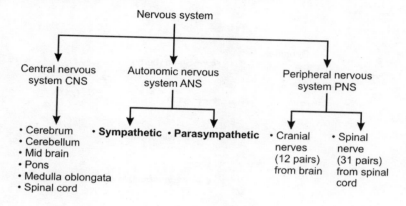

As per Function

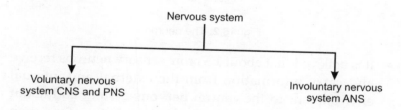

As per Location

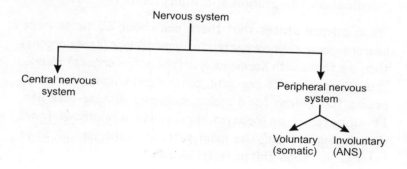

CENTRAL NERVOUS SYSTEM

1. *Cerebral hemispheres:* **Planning the movement:**
   - Also called as big brain. Two in number, right and left brain.
   - Both have varied functions to perform other than motor control.
   - They have contralateral control of the motor functions of body.
   - Right brain is the feminine brain. It is sensitive and has creative aspect.
   - Left brain is the masculine brain. It is logical and has rational aspect
   - Each hemisphere is divided into four lobes, all of them having different functions to perform. It is beyond the scope of this book to go into its details.

"Yoga believes that (with neurophysiological investigation) when one breathes with left nostril, right side of brain activities are controlled, whereas when one breathes through right nostril, the left brain function are controlled. When one holds the breath (as in Kumbhaka phase of Pranayama) both the hemispheres become active and operative, and increase alertness and awareness to carry out any motor task. These experiences demonstrate, the significant effect of Pranayama, specially Anulom vilom Pranayama, the alternate nostril breath for controlling flow of breath, through which deeper structures of brain can regain mental, emotional and physical equilibrium."

2. *Basal ganglia:* **Programming and regulating the movement:**
   - It is mainly responsible for **postural fixation facilitation** through extrapyramidal system on fusimotor system of stretch reflex mechanism via reticular formation.

- It **regulates** rhythmic free movements of distal components of body.
- It regulates reflex activities.
- It is responsible for adequate necessary malleability of voluntary movements and associated reactions.

"Yogic practise of Asanas, specifically Sarvangasana (shoulder stand posture) and Bhujangasana (Cobra posture) facilitate postural fixation through the above stated mechanism.

Regular practise of Anulom vilom Pranayama helps in regulating rate and rhythm of movements by balancing the dopamine, acetylecholine synthesis."

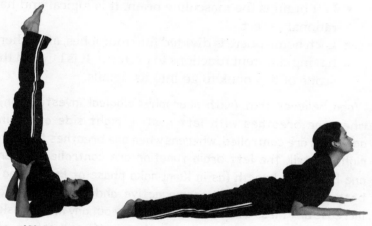

(A) Modified Sarvangasana   **(B)** Bhujangasana

Figs 16.3A and B: Asana and movement regulation

3. *Thalamus:* **Awareness of movement**
   - All types of sensory feelings reach this area first.
   - It helps for awareness, alertness and consciousness.
   - It has a role to play for emotional balance, specially in "pain."

"Regular and sincere practice of the Ashtangyoga ladder in day to day life sequences has a very positive role to play in prevention and elimination of all painful syndromes—Mental and Physical. It increases pain tolerance capacity of an individual."

4. *Hypothalamus:* **Regulation and control of the functional movement:**
   - It is the important part of the brain and is concerned with homeostasis of body.
   - Regulates many vital functions of the body like endocrine, visceral through ANS, metabolic activities, hunger, thirst, sleep, wakefulness, emotions and sexual functions.

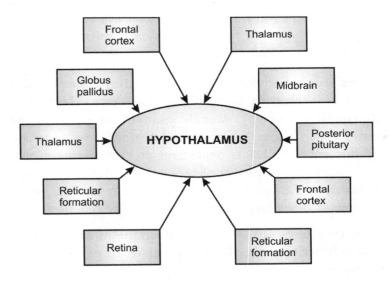

Fig. 16.4: Connections of Hypothalamus

- It also regulates temperature, blood pressure and heart rate.
- Emotional changes and behaviour are also controlled by it.
- It is the regulating centre for many ANS activities and functioning.

- It is also called as "Biological clock" and controls activities like:
  - Menstrual cycle
  - Fluctuation of temperature
  - Fluctuation in hormonal level.

"Yoga science believes that "**stress**"—Physical and Mental causes Hypothalmic overactivation involving immune system and autonomic activation (Mind body disorders)."

"Overactivation of these two systems of defence mechanism of body, lowers the stress coping mechanism of body which eventually gives rise to all conversion physical symptoms (Psychosomatic disorders)."

"Yogic practise of the 8 steps explained by Sage Patanjali helps in inculcating Social discipline (Yama), Individual discipline (Niyama), Muscle relaxation and Energy conservation (Asanas), Breath regulation and oxygen storage as this part of CNS is dependent on rich oxygen supply (Pranayama], Lifestyle discipline (Pratyahara) and Meditation (Dhyana) increase chemical liberation of neuropeptides, which have mood regulating and emotional stability functions."

"This improves stress coping mechanism and immune system function, prevents and reverses all psychosomatic disorders."

5. *Lymbic system*

- It is the organ of movement synchronisation, regulation, co-ordination, etc.
- It is an important centre of emotion, memory and olfaction.
- Emotion consists of analysis:

   a. *Cognition:* means seeing and recognising

   b. *Affect:* means development of feeling

c. *Conation:* means desire to act

d. *Expression:* means the act/response.

- Personality of an individual is formed of these three aspects:

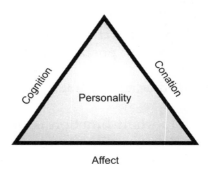

Fig. 16.5: The three aspects of personality

- As the person uses the sense organs **(cognition)**, so does the feeling and emotion **(affect)** develops. Based on his ability and knowledge to perceive he acts and reacts to these emotions **(conation)**.

"Yogic science believes that with the knowledge of the controlled use of the sense organs, withdrawing oneself from distracting stimuli of the sense organs (Pratyahaar), one can maintain mind body harmony."

"Sitting in a comfortable position, eyes closed and concentrating on "Ajna chakra" or pineal gland through breath regulation is one of the "relaxing techniques."

"Yogic science considers the secretion of pineal gland as "Chandramrut" or "Melatonin" which is soothening and tranquilising to the mind. Increase in this secretion gives one a feeling of well being and he experiences full consciousness of joy of life."

"This is a very effective means in Rehabilitation of Stroke and Parkinsonism syndrome patients, as it can calm down the emotions. Disease may not be cured, but emotions can be calmed down."

6. *Cerebellum:* **Decides movement tactics**
   - They have ipsilateral control of the body. *Also called as small brain, two is number-right and left.*
   - A main organ of postural tone, balance and equilibrium.
   - It is also called as a comparator and error correcting mechanism.
   - Its other important function is of muscular co-ordination.
   - To my knowledge, no much research has been reported in curative aspect of Yogic practise of cerebellar disorders.

"Yogic practise of Pranayama and Meditation can strengthen and improve the immune system of an individual and prevent autoimmune disorders that can affect cerebellum."

7. *Spinal Cord:* **Execution of the movement**
   - It is the connecting organ between the higher and middle order neural tissue of CNS with the peripheral neural tissues (PNS).
   - It is the centre that executes the movement planned by the central cortex through motor neuronal pool (lower motor neuron).
   - It carries sensations from the periphery, of pain, touch, temperature, bladder and bowel fullness.
   - Adjustments and selective movements patterns are decided, executed and also process of defaecation is performed normally through it.
   - The spinal level reflex activity is controlled here which allows all the types of movement patterns to be performed precisely and as per the demands, commanded for the task.

"With Yogic practise, research has stated that the intra-neuronal activity in spinal cord (intermediate area between the anterior and posterior horns of grey matter) is benefited, as they are responsible for processing the incoming sensory information from periphery, as well as descending signals from higher brain centres."

"Pranayama facilitates the Alpha motor neuron activity as they are responsible for postural adjustments and adaptations (alpha motor neuron supplies skeletal muscle fibres)"

"Pranayama and Meditation also have inhibiting influences to control the over-excitation of muscle contraction in pyramidal pathway lesion. This aspect can prevent spastic contractures to develop in the affected muscles and make it easy for these patients to carry out their daily functional tasks for rehabilitation in all aspects of their living."

THE AUTONOMIC NERVOUS SYSTEM

- It is also called as involuntary nervous system, controlling and regulating the functions of visceral organs.
- This system has two components that have functionally antagonistic roles, the sympathetic and the parasympathetic.
- Under normal circumstances, however, both work in a synchronised pattern.
- It overall controls autonomic reflexes like:
  - Arterial blood pressure.
  - Heart rate and rhythm.
  - Gastro-intestinal mobility and secretions.
  - Urinary bladder filling and emptying.
  - Sweating.
  - Body temperature.

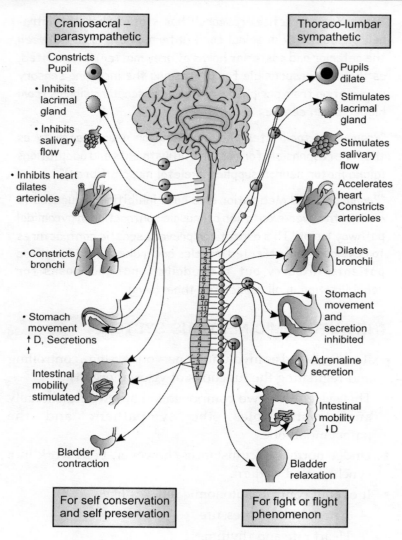

Fig. 16.6: The autonomic nervous system

- It is under the control of subconscious mind, the functions of which are to think, to feel, to behave, etc. Anything that causes emotional disturbances, affects the synergistic activity balance of these two components.

- If there is sympathetic imbalance then symptoms generally related with **coronary artery disease, hypertension, CV stroke, etc. develop.**
- If there is parasympathetic imbalance then symptoms usually related to **bronchial asthama, irritable bowel syndrome, etc. develop.**

"Hath Yoga classifies the
    Sympathetic as male energy—'Ha', and
    Parasympathetic as female energy—'Tha'

Balance of these two energies maintains balance and harmony between mind and body, preventing health problems and maintaining positive health.

Anulom vilom Pranayama, the alternate nostril breathing is one of the methods to balance these energies, if practised with dedication sincerity and regularity. A sense of inner peace and relaxation is felt when a state of equilibrium is reached.

Concentration on the Yogic chakras, the centres of generation and regulation of these energies also helps in harmonising these two systems, and achieve a state of homeostasis.

PERIPHERAL NERVOUS SYSTEM

- They are bundle of axons, conducting efferent (motor) impulse from centre (anterior horn cells) of spinal cord to the muscles, and afferent (sensory) impulses from periphery to the centre (posterior horn cells) of spinal cord.
- They may be affected by disease, damage or degeneration.

"Yogic practise of Asanas specifically the Cultural Asanas benefit in improving the conduction pathway transmission by re-conditioning of the spinal nerves through the improved vascularity effect of the Asanas. Symptoms of radiculities and radiculopathy are reduced and overcome by the regular practise."

"The reflex activity control is also facilitated which improves the stretch reflex perceptibility and hence prevents stress and strain falling on these neural tissues."

"Yogasana like Vajrasana, Paadhasthasana, Mastyasana through proprioceptive neuromuscular stimulation facilitate stretch reflex activity and improve vascularity of these spinal nerves."

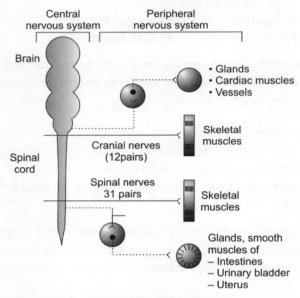

Fig. 16.7: The peripheral nervous system

Asana beneficial to peripheral nervous system functioning are:

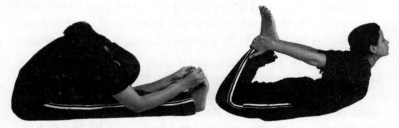

(A) Paschimottanasana   **(B)** Dhanurasana—The bow pose

Figs 16.8A and B: Asana beneficial on peripheral nervous system

- These Asanas should be practised after appropriate assessment and under guidance of an expert.
- Overcoming this debilitating and frustrating problem of neuralgias and sciatica, make the rehabilitation plan and process worth following with interest and ease.

GOALS OF PHYSICAL THERAPY

1. **Assess** thoroughly the severity of symptoms caused by the neurological disturbances, since their effect can be considerably alleviated by proper therapy and guidelines.
2. **Restore** the maximum functional ability, so that the patient can be an integral functional part of the family, society and community in terms of economical status too.
3. **Reduce** incapacitating symptoms of tonal abnormalities.
4. **Train** faculties left to the patient to compensate for the lost ones.
5. **Prevent** all secondary complications.
6. **Educate** and **encourage** the patient to accept and live with his disability with courage and zeal.

MY BELIEFS AND VIEWS ON NEURO-DISORDERS' APPROACH: AS A PHYSIOTHERAPIST AND A YOGA TEACHER

- Qualitative assessment of a function is a pre-requisite for assessment and improvement of motor control rather than quantitative measures of grading **(wholistic view).**
- The ability of function normally depends upon the patient's ability to the demands of the environment, and to his own needs quickly, efficiently and effectively. The ability to achieve this state depends on the availability of the mature nervous system with healthy functioning **(wholistic outlook).**

- Every movement begins in a posture and ends in a posture. Posture and movement are so closely related that it is impossible to distinguish one from the other. Cephalocaudal pattern of development should be kept in mind as a framework for assessment, guideline and management **(wholistic assessment)**.

- A patient with neurological deficit usually shows:
  - Poverty of movement synergy.
  - Regression of motor skill.
  - Disturbance of balance reaction.
  - Abnormal posturing.

- Hence:
  - It is a great mistake to wait till the patient is conscious.
  - Early intervention should be prime requisite.
  - Normal sequence of development ladder to be followed.
  - One should not go on hunting for the disabilities, but should find out abilities left in the patient and encourage and strengthen his will power and morale.
  - Rehabilitation of all aspects should be kept in mind **(wholistic approach)**.

1. Bobath's Neurodevelopmental Technique and Yogasana

- The NDT approach focuses on postures and movement that inhibits abnormal tone and abnormal reflex activity and encourages postures that promote and facilitate normal movement.

- This abnormal reflex activity is due to loss or affection in the inhibiting pathways that control the postural tone and movements.

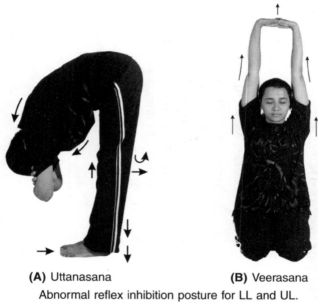

(A) Uttanasana   **(B)** Veerasana

Abnormal reflex inhibition posture for LL and UL.

Figs 16.9A and B: Asana and Bobath's NDT postures

- Key point of control: Spine
- Mind-body approach facilitate relearning process.
- Bilateral limbs activity approach.

"Yogic practise is self-analysis, self-commanding and self-error correction technique."

Table 16.1: Yogic practice and NDT

The aspects of NDT	The aspects of Yogic posture
• Proper positioning of head and neck	• Erect spine: The basic requirement
• Weight bearing facilitates postural tone through joint approximation.	• Standing Asana Tadasana: It strengthen postural mechanisms.
• Trunk rotation inhibits overactive stretch reflex activity.	• Twisting Asana Vakrasana: Focuses on spinal rotation, for movement control.
• Scapular and pelvic protraction position encouraged for ADL.	• All asana emphasize on Shoulder and Pelvic girdle strengthening, for ADL.
• Facilitation of slow, controlled movement.	• The process of 'going into and release' of Asana should be slow, rhythmic act
• Commands to be followed with concentration	• Asana is Psychophysical posture hence, Autocommands favours concentration

2. Movement Control: Rajyoga Ladder

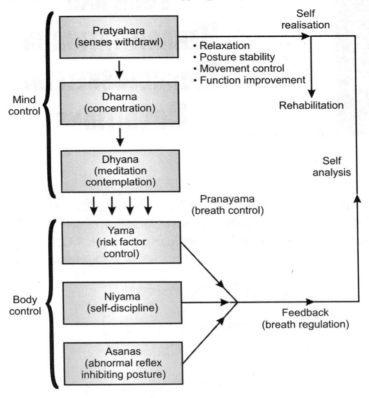

Mind → body control : Stroke rehabilitation
Parkinsonian syndromes
Ataxias (cerabellar)

Fig. 16.10: Movement control Patanjali's Rajyoga ladder

The effects of mind-body control technique explained in Fig. 16.10 can achieve relaxation, postural stability, movement control and functions improvement, which can aid in functional rehabilitation of CV stroke, Parkinson's and Ataxic patients.

SUMMARY

1. Yogic practice has a multi faceted approch for patient of neuro muscular disorder. The scerect of rehabilitation is to give right help at right time.

<table>
<tr><td rowspan="2" style="writing-mode: vertical">Chapter</td><td rowspan="2">17</td><td># YOGA AND REHABILITATION IN MUSCULOSKELETAL CONDITIONS</td></tr>
</table>

YOGA AND REHABILITATION IN MUSCULOSKELETAL CONDITIONS

Chapter 17

"Sometimes we must be HURT in order to GROW, we must FALL in order to KNOW, we must LOOSE in order to GAIN, because some lessons are best learnt through PAIN."

— A Quotable Quote.

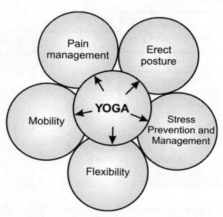

Fig. 17.1: Applications of Yoga

- Musculoskeletal pain disorders have reached epidemic proportions all over and have been a great challenge to all professionals dealing in its prevention and elimination.

"Pain needs to be understood more as a feeling than a mere sensation."

- Many books, great discussions, various symposiums, good texts, chapters, paragraphs have been in circulation and enormous efforts have been put up by professionals each day to combat this agonising problem. However, many write-ups, therapies, surgical interventions, bracings and medicines have been suggested, advocated and implemented worldwide for pain-relief. Here, in this Chapter I have focussed on the role of psychosocial factors as one of the main contributors to these painful syndromes.

MY DOUBTS, CURIOSITIES AND CONCERN

- Why day-by-day this agonising problem is increasing despite of medical advancement?
- Why every two years a new modality is introduced in physiotherapy for pain relief?
- Why the patients have recurrence of pain inspite of being under best medical and physiotherapy care?
- The answer that I Feel is worth giving attention to is to **Stress—Physical and Mental**.
- The remedy, the solution, the relief measure that I Feel to the problem is "The SELF."
- The philosophy

  The word Human Being where "Human" means "external framework of bone and flesh."

  "Being" means "the invisible power within."

  The well being of this skeletal of bone and flesh is strengthened by the invisible power within "The SELF."

  The acceptance of this "Self" as a motivator and manager of pain works faster and with long-lasting result than any other *"pathies and therapies"* in relieving oneself from this problem.

THE PSYCHO-BIOMECHANICAL OUTLOOK

- Our body is a living machine functioning in accordance with the universal laws of motion and its mechanical principles. It is an intricate structure of bones, muscles, ligaments, capsule and joints with the amazing versatility of movements it can perform.
- The muscles of our body cannot only pull but can also push, lift, strike, throw, kick, walk, run, jump and are capable of many more functions. To perform all these activities efficiency of movement is very important.
- The efficiency depends on amount of work done and force of energy expended. In human motion, it is the ratio of external work accomplished to the muscle energy spent.
- Whenever there is an imbalance between the demand of the body and the supply of energy in form of muscular work, the normal body alignment changes, causing stress and strain in one or the other parts of the segments of the body resulting into various musculoskeletal problems with the most common complain of **PAIN.**
- Today with great advancements which have been made in medicine, both in diagnostic and therapeutic fields, it is essential that all who deal with patients on the road to recovery from this agonising problem should be equipped **with a clear understanding of the cause, mechanism and approach of treatment which they offer.**

THE PSYCHOSOMATIC FACTOR

- The worry about the **future**, the **present** state of anxiety due to pain and the apprehension about the **past** adds to the severity of pain experience and aggravates the physical symptoms.
- The **Mental stress** that accumulates within reflects in physical responses like disturbed or weak postural

mechanisms and muscular tensions which cause fatigue postures and put loading stress on all weight bearing joints leading to musculo-skeletal postural problems.

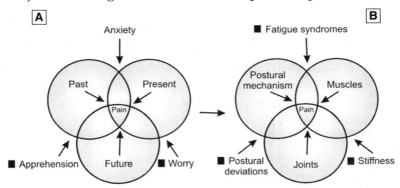

Figs. 17.2A and B: (A) The psyche role **(B)** The soma response

- **Negative emotions** like Fear, Rage, Anxiety, Hatred, Frustration, Worry, Anger, Jealousy, Apprehension and many such emotions generate tension in the muscles through Autonomic nervous system imbalance and if this persists for a long-time then it, causes poor vascularity, tissue hypoxia and **fatigue syndromes**.

- *Eventually as postural deviations develop, energy consumption increases, uneven loading stress falls on the joints like knee, intervertebra and ankle joints aggravating the pathophysiological changes.*

- The centre of pain perception and emotions are mutually affected in the **limbic system** in the brain.

  - Positive emotions give positive perception and increase pain tolerance.

  - Negative emotions give negative perception and decrease pain tolerance.

"The Self Concept Experience" of severity of pain is a very subjective issue and varies from person to person and this is what YOGA explains and guides.

THE ASSOCIATED PSYCHOSOMATIC DISORDERS

- **Assessment of the cause of disturbance** of musculoskeletal system needs more specification and attention rather than **routine physical assessment criteria of Range of motion, Muscle power, Postural alterations, Deformities,** etc. as, all these are secondarily affected in these conditions.

- **Examining the other causes** which could have altered the posture is also essential. These causes could be due to:
  - Emotions and personality traits.
  - Respiratory system problems.
  - Cardiovascular system problems.
  - Neural problems.
  - Viscerogenic problems.
  - Habitual factors like faulty body mechanics and ergonomics in activities of daily living.

- All these can also be the root cause of painful syndromes or could be the triggering or aggravating factors.

- Evidences, Research and Experience have confirmed that musculoskeletal problems have been increasing in recent time due to **stress, stressors** and **poor stress coping mechanisms**, may it be accidental injuries, traumatic injuries, or pain of non-specific origin.

- Stress and pre-occupied thoughts lead to accidents as a result of weakening of all reflex activities specifically the **protective reflex**. Cause of musculoskeletal involvement is no doubt the accident, but the reason for the cause is "the disturbed psyche."

- **Repressed rage,** as research states is also one of the instigating factor of Painful syndromes. **Accumulated rage results due to lack of communication and no proper outlet of emotions.** This triggers sympathetic nervous system overactivity, muscular tension, impaired vascularity, reduced oxygen supply, tissue hypoxia, increased level of lactic acid deposition and PAIN.

"A transformational change is necessary rather than conventional methods of assessment and treatment"

"Self transformation leads to transformation of any situation"

THE RATIONALE OF PHYSIOTHERAPY IS

1. **To harmonise** all the body segments with each other by physical means like remedial exercise, soft tissue mobilisations, manipulative techniques, relaxation methods, hydrotherapy, cryotherapy, electrotherapy, etc. as per the requirements so as **to restore and improve the musculo skeletal framework back to normal.**

2. **To restore the rights, previlege and reputation of the patient,** so that he becomes an integral and functional part of family and society.

3. **To conserve energy with economy** of effort by application of techniques based on biomechanical principles.

4. **To avoid strain and prevent structural changes** to occur by appropriate Ergonomic advices.

5. **To encourage and achieve economical and functional independence.**

The above goals can be fulfilled more competently with the patient's participation positively, willingly, dedicatedly and with sincerity **(self-analysis).** The target can be achieved faster with the patient's good mental endurance, functional breathing patterns, alert reflex mechanism and good perceptual function. **The road to recovery can be enhanced with Yogic practise.**

"Physiotherapy is the means, Yoga is the path."

ASHTANGYOGA AND PAIN RELIEF

1. Yama-Niyama and Pain Relief

- Introducing and inculcating **core values within oneself,** changes the outlook for pain and brings a quality change to understand the problem.
- Values with **good deeds** (Karmas) have tremendous power in healing.
- Values also empower the immune system and strengthen coping mechanisms and reduce stress levels, mental and physical.
- Acceptance of pain as "A part of life" and following the **ergonomic advices** with sincerity and simplicity in lifestyle help to recover faster.

"Yama (social discipline) and Niyama (individual discipline) form the foundation for pain relief programme."

2. Yogasanas and Pain Relief

- It is a **psychophysical posture** where mind-body concentration is must.
- The dynamic component of the Asana strengthens the **musculoskeletal** framework and the static component relaxes the **neuromuscular framework**.
- **Regular practise** of Asanas achieves good health, keeping body in good shape, psyche fit and relaxed so as to cope with various turbulences of life and not fall prey to psychosomatic painful disorders.
- Relaxation Asanas like Balkasana and Makarasan can be practised by anyone with any type of painful syndrome.

- Cultural Asanas (for health) should be selectively practised for therapeutic purpose, under the proper supervision and guidance.
- The Asanas that can be practised by all irrespective of some associated problems are:

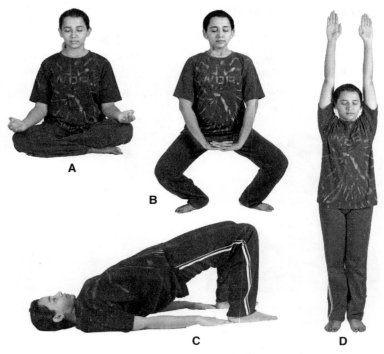

(A) Sukhasana (B) Utthitasana (C) Setubandhasana
(D) Modified Tadasana

Figs 17.3A to D: Yogasanas and pain relief

The advantages of Asanas for pain relief

1. **Relaxes** the muscles and **relieves** muscular tension.
2. **Regulates** the breath and **increases** pain tolerance.
3. **Lubricates** the joints and **reduces** painful stiffness.
4. **Improves** pliability of soft tissues around joints.
5. **Strengthens** the antigravity mechanism for erect posture.

6. Reduces the levels of **blood lactate** and prevents fatigueness.

7. **Reconditions** the peripheral nerves thereby **improving** pain perception.

3. Pranayama and Pain Relief

- Food, water and air are basic elements on which human being survives. Of the three, **air is said to be the vital source of energy.**
- As good the storage and conservation of this energy, better will be the cellular nutrition and health.

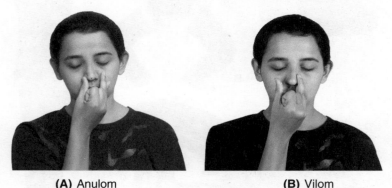

(A) Anulom   **(B)** Vilom
Figs 17.4A and B: Pranayama and pain relief

- If breath is life then, it is essential that the air we breath should be fresh, pure and **adequately oxygenated.**
- Purification of all the channels is the keynote of Hathyoga and fore most practise of purification is **Pranayama**.
- The mind benefits from calming and toning of nervous system, and tone and texture of nervous system are influenced by the rate and rhythm of respiration.
- Pranayama that can be practised safely by anyone with painful syndrome:

- **Anulom-vilom** also called as "Nadi Shodhan" for purification of channels and mind-body balance.
- **Ujjayi,** the victorious breath for relaxation purpose.

The Advantages of Pranayama for Pain Relief

1. **Energises** and **exercises** the lungs and **improves** vital capacity.
2. **Aids** good vascularity and oxygenation to the tissues.
3. **Soothes** and **tones** the nerves.
4. **Improves** thoracic mobility and abdominal muscle tone.
5. **Trains** the diaphragm, thoracic and abdominal muscles to operate effectively in all activities of daily living.
6. The *"bandhs"* or "locks" like **Uddiyan** and **Jalandhar** **strengthen** and **stabilise** the lumbar and cervical spine.
7. The *"mool bandh"* or "perineal lock "**strengthen** the pelvic floor muscles and is a great means to enhance women's health in all age groups.

"Judicious practise of Pranayam attains sound health, slim and lustrous posture and peaceful pain free body."

4. Meditation and Pain Relief

Meditation: Mastery Over Attention: A – Tension

- Recent belief about *"meditation being the best method of Relaxation"* is gaining great popularity.
- It develops a feeling of "self worth" and balances all aspects of personality and channelises all systems too. This aspect takes care of the root cause of the painful syndrome and **helps in alleviating the responsible psychosocial factor of pain.**

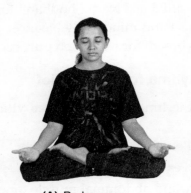 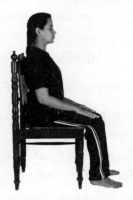

(A) Padmasana   **(B)** The Chairpose

Figs 17.5A and B: Meditation poses and pain relief

- It replaces the feeling of negativity with the feeling of happiness, contentment and openness. The outlook and attitude towards life changes. One follows the command of "Self" and modifies lifestyle patterns, food habits willingly and becomes his own manager.
- **Breath watching meditation** or Concentration on **"Ajna chakra"** (between the eyebrows) or Pineal gland is believed to be effective means of meditation for pain relief. **Calming the mind calms the body.**
- Regular practise of meditation in any comfortable position for 10 to 15 minutes in a day can be best psychotherapeutic technique in the management programme for pain relief.

5. The Yogic Advice and Pain Relief

    a. No "don'ts" and only "do's" as advice.

    b. Resume physical activity as early as possible. It helps.

    c. In non-specific pain, discontinue all physical treatments. They may be blocking the recovery. (Conditioning Response)

    d. Be aware of the "stressors" but ignore them slowly and steadily.

e. Be frank, free, flexible and always fresh in communication.

f. Listen to all, but believe in yourself.

g. Eat fresh food, breathe fresh air and drink plenty of water.

h. Practise Yogasana regularly and rhythmically as adviced.

i. Ergonomic advice of lifting, carrying, bending, sitting standing, etc. to be followed as adviced.

6. The Diet and Pain Relief

Table 17.1: The yogic diet and pain relief

Food to be avoided	Food allowed
• Cold refrigerated drinks and dishes.	• Fresh cooked food.
• Sour and bitter food.	• Milk and its products.
• Hot and spicy food.	• Honey and sugars.
• Fried food items.	• Mild spices, ginger, garlic.
• Alcohol and other beverages.	• Warm soups.
• Refined cereals.	• Whole grains.
• Preservative and processed food.	• Limited quantities of fats and oils.
• Non-vegetarian food.	• Vegetarian food with green vegetable.
• Citrus fruits like orange and its types	• All types of pulp fruits.

7. The Lifestyle and Pain Relief

• An integrated **biologically clocked lifestyle** to be followed.

• The proverb **"Early to bed early to rise, makes a person healthy wealthy and wise"** holds true.

• The Rajyoga saying, **"Soil is everything seed is nothing."**

• The common sense: Sensible footwear and clothing.

• The guidelines: Regularity in activities of daily living.

• The physiotherapist's advice: The programme should be followed only after **thorough biomechanical assessment.**

THE INTEGRATED APPROACH

As per the explanation and content of preceding chapters of Yoga and Biomechanics, and Yoga and Exercise Therapy the following analysis can be made for the management programme of approximately all the musculoskeletal problems.

Table 17.2: The integrated approach and pain relief

Aim	Physical therapy	Yogic practise
a. Stability	• Close kinematic chain exercise	• The Yogic posture 'Asana'
b. Mobility	• Open kinematic chain exercise	• Sukshmakriyas
c. Strength	• Principles of strengthening	• Dynamic state of Asana
d. Endurance	• Rhythmic stabilisation	• Asana and Dharna
e. Tissue nourishment	• Breathing exercise	• Pranayama
f. Erect posture	• Postural exercise	• Asana and Pranayam
g. Relaxation	• JPMR, Hold-Relax, Reciprocal relaxation techniques	• All the seven steps of Rajyoga ladder

THE MUSCULOSKELETAL CONDITIONS BENEFITTED BY THE INTEGRATED APPROACH

- All back and neck problems
- Shoulder arm complex problems
- Knee problems
- Planter fascities
- Tennis elbow
- Sciatica and other neuralgias
- Rheumatoid arthritis.

SUMMARY

1. The combination of Sukshmakriyas (the Yogic warm up) Yogasana (pain gate control mechanism) Pranayama (Relaxation) and Dhyana-meditation (Harmonisation of mind body) conserves mental and physical energies.

2. The integration **clarifies** the Physical self, **educates** the mind and body, **co-ordinates** the Psyche and Soma, **inculcates** self-confidence and energy conservation thereby achieving **Pain Relief**.

3. Not reacting to painful syndromes but,
   - **Observe** the aggravating factors.
   - **Listen** to the body signals.
   - **Understand** the relieving factors.
   - **Analyse** the difference.
   - **Perform** the task with confidence.

The above, will certainly help in preventing and alleviating musculoskeletal problems.

YOGA AND WOMEN'S HEALTH

"The ability to educate women about the role of exercise and health promotion provides a significant professional opportunity and responsibility"

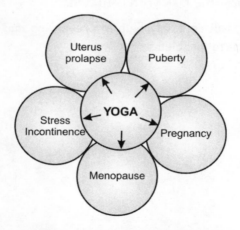

Fig. 18.1: Women's health and Yoga applications

- During the growth and development phase of a woman, tremendous *physical, mental* and *hormonal changes* take place and yet she is to be in a state of wellness always.

IS TODAY'S WOMAN STRESSED ???

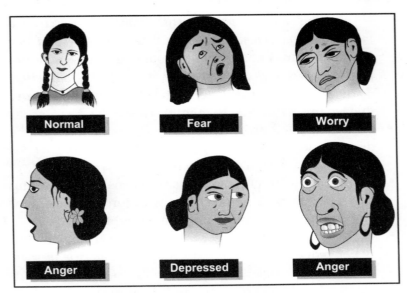

Fig. 18.2: Women in stress

- Lifestyle, food habits, modern gadgets, dual role of a home maker and a professional, family expectations, work place demands, etc. all have been *stressors* to a woman.
- *Sedentary life* affects the larger population of women in India.
- *Modern day lifestyle* also has affected women with many *postural problems, joint pathomechanics, pain syndromes, etc.*
- *Food habits* further more have contributed to increase in the problems.
- *Mental stress* is the greatest agonizing problem for women today due to the imbalance between the role expectations and the performance levels.

Stress does Not have to be All Bad...

- The *short term* effects of high level stress can cause *fatigue, sleeplessness, anxiety, poor appetite, headache, backache and many other conversion problems.* If this continues for *a long time* then it may contribute to potentially serious health problems like *high blood pressure, diabetes, gastrointestinal disturbances and ulcers.* **Research has reported many gynaec problems due to mental stress.**
- When managed properly, stress can provide us with the drive to meet new challenges. It is ony when *stress builds up to uncomfortable level, it can be harmful.*
- Confidence with consequent easing of tension and settling down of internal rhythm comes with fore knowledge of how to deal with any situation that might arise.
- When a woman knows how to help herself and co-operate as per requested, *how to relax or exert her muscle in right way and right time, the whole process of her life during* ***Menarche, Menstruation and Menopause becomes smoother and much more satisfactory.***
- Since emotional tension leads to physical tension, it is of prime importance for her to *learn **relaxation methods,*** as it is one of the important aspect in the dimension for a ***blessed womanhood.***

"Women should be respected in all her avatars (roles) as a mother, as a daughter, as a sister, and as a wife."

YOGA FOR WOMEN IN ALL HER AVATARS (ROLES)

- *Yoga* blesses women with *charm, elegance, beauty and suppleness.*
- *Yoga tranquilises* the mind, *relaxes* the muscles, *mobilizes* the joints, *regulates* her breath thereby regulating her life to take charge of her roles bestowed upon her with dignity and poise.

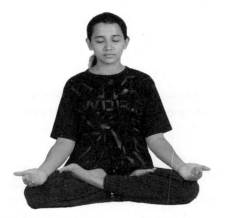

Fig. 18.3: Yoga for women—Padmasana

- *Yogic practise* also helps in *controlling and reducing fat deposition in the areas prone to it.*
- It *relieves mental fatigue* in women, thereby preventing premature physical changes of aging.
- *Yoga* helps in *prenatal programming of brain function of foetus* also, thereby maintaining *vigour and vitality throughout life of both, the mother and child.*
- Yoga also helps to reduce and *prevent Perinatal problem* due to stress like spontaneous abortion, structural malformation, preterm delivery and decreased birth weight.
- *Yoga* also takes care of *Postnatal functions* of woman if there are problems like high blood pressure, migraine, postural imbalances, anxiety disorders, cardiovascular disorder, etc.
- *Yoga* also helps *prevent transmission of maternal stress* to the unborn baby by increased blood flow to uterus and foetus and *increasing parasympathetic balance and functioning.*

- *Yoga and Yogic practise uplift and strengthen the woman's morale and functioning, mentally and physically during the menopause phase,* leading her to accept mind, body and life situation with positivism and zeal.

"Yoga improves optimism in all life situation of woman, keeping her stress level under control for effective functioning always."

THE APPROACH

- Today medical science has advanced in an astonishing way. Knowledge of science enables one to solve even the most complicated issues.
- The Therapist is able to assess and monitor the physical changes, musculoskeletal functioning, emotional balance and accordingly enhance the motivational level, learning skills, adaptation and adjustment levels with the primary focus in maintaining wellness at all stages. **One of the important aspects in this dimension is maintaining pelvic floor health** for an uncomplicated pregnancy, easy labour, cheerful motherhood and blessed womanhood.
- The great Maharshi Patanjali, the father of Yogic practise quotes that "changes can occur in the genes and the enviroment in the whole human system by regular and sincere practise of Dharna (Concentration) and Dhyana (Meditation). These Yoga practises are non invasive, economical, easy to perform, culturally acceptable and pleasant means to healthy lifestyle mentally and physically.
- The Integrated Approach with thorough Biomechanical assessment of musculoskeletal framework, cardio-respiratory endurance, and neuromuscular functioning by the therapist along with the Wholistic guidelines and management in Yogic way, take care of women's issues successfully.

THE ISSUES

1. Menstruation

- Yoga has an enriching effect on the hormonal system balance and functioning that will help relieve symptoms of pre-menstrual pain (PMS) and generally will keep one healthier, fresh, and full of energy during this phase.
- One should not practise Yogasanas during the days of heaviest bleeding.
- One may do simple stretching warm ups but avoid anything that compresses the abdominal area either in forward or backward positioning.
- **Yama** (social discipline) should be followed to avoid conflicts in day to day situations to take care of the emotional changes that occur with menstruation.
- **Niyama** (individual discipline) of personal hygiene good reading, sensible footwear and clothing during this phase if is followed then discomfort and uneasiness will be less.
- Yogasanas that are beneficial during this phase are:
  - Uttanasana   – Parvatasana
  - Veerasana   – Upvistakonasana

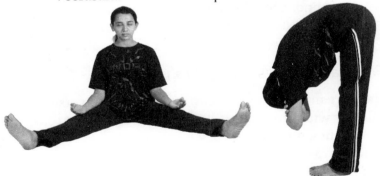

(A) Modified—Upvistakonasana   (B) Uttanasana

Figs 18.4A and B: Asana during menstruation

- **Pranayama** that can be practised during this cycle: Anulom vilom in any comfortable sitting posture.
- **Dharna or concentration on Swadhistan Chakra**–the perineal region for 10-15 minutes also helps in relieving from pelvic congestion discomfort feeling.

2. Pregnancy

- Pregnancy is a straight forward, happy and healthy time for a woman. If this time is nourished, cared, comforted with appropriate psychological, physiological and social support system then both the mother and child become a functional integral and productive part of society and can make their own rehabilitation easy after the delivery.
- Pregnancy is a special time for a woman and her family. It is a time of many changes in the pregnant woman's body and her emotions. These changes add new stresses to the life as demand increases physically emotionally and socially.
- The pregnant woman is nourishing a dynamic life within her hence she should be approached with wholistic care. According to Yoga **"Moderation is the key."** This programme makes the:
  - mind calm, peaceful and happy.
  - gives stamina and vitality to the body.
  - promotes positive health of mother and child both.

Physical Changes During Pregnancy

There are many changes occurring which are reversible after delivery with proper care.

- Weight gain as pregnancy progresses.
- Respiratory discomforts like breathlessness and dyspnoea.
- Fatigue and exhaustion due to increase oxygen consumption.

- Cardiovascular changes like increased blood pressure, heart rate, pedel oedema.
- Muscular and ligamentous laxity due to hormonal changes and foetal growth.
- Postural imbalances due to altered centre of gravity.
- Postural disorders like exaggerated lordosis due to sagging shoulders (breast enlargement and foetal growth).

Emotional Changes During Pregnancy

- A Feeling of insecurity and nervousness.
- Sometimes one feels depressed and low due to physiological changes.
- Is always in need of assurance and motivation.
- Loss of appetite.

"The materialistic way of lifestyle has lost all faith in spirituality."

The Yogic Practise During Pregnancy

Startling new research states that adult illnesses like diabetes, obesity, asthma, hypertension, etc. may have their roots before birth.

- Documented research in Yoga therapy states that there are beneficial effects of Yoga in PREGNANCY.
- There are many books written in Yoga for pregnant women, describing the practises and help in relaxed pregnancy and easy delievery.
- Yogic practise if started before the conception itself, nurtures baby's overall growth and development at the physical, mental, emotional and intellectual capacities.
- Practise of Yoga effectively awakens the Prana-the vital source of energy, in foetus which may cause various unusual movements of energy in body and mind (Quickening movement of foetus in IInd trimester).

- Yogic practise during pregnancy should be followed under care and supervision of an expert. It
  - Maintains a well developed and normally shaped pelvis.
  - Maintains flexibility in joints of pelvis and lower limbs.
  - Maintains an unconstrained attitude for pregnancy, and delivery.
  - Eradicates all fears and tensions of woman and builds confidence.
- Yogic exercise can also be called as **"Psychoprophylaxia"** which emphasis two aspects.
  - **Reconditioning** of woman's psyche to remove pain associated with child birth.
  - **Concentration** technique which blocks the painful stimuli and improve pain threshold for easy labour.

Therapeutic Effects of Yogic Exercise

1. *The relaxation asanas:* Takes care of stress, pain and muscle imbalance from faulty posture.
2. Develops awareness and control of posture during and after pregnancy by strengthening the postural mechanisms – The Cultural Asana-*Upvistakonasana.*
3. Develops upper extremity strength for the demands of infant care with Asanas like *Setubandhasana* (Bridging) and *Anulom-vilom breathing*.
4. Prepares the lower extremities for the demands of increased weight bearing and circulatory compromise- Lower limb *Sukshmakriyas* for mobility. Weight bearing standing Asana like *Tadasana* (Fundamental standing posture) and *Setubandhasana.*
5. Develops awareness and control of pelvic floor muscles. *Mool bandh or perineal lock-a psychophysical form of Kegel's exercise.*

6. Maintains and strengthens abdominal function in antenatal and postnatal phase with all Asanas, expiratory phase of Pranayama and *Uddiyan bandh* (abdominal lock).

7. Promotes and maintains safe cardiovascular and cardio-respiratory fitness with *Pranayama , Dharna and Dhyana*.

8. Learn relaxation skills (relaxation Asana-modified *Shavasana* posture).

9. Prevent and overcome all pathologies induced by pregnancy by mental relaxation (*Pratyahara, Dharna and Dhyana*).

"Yogic practise controls, guides and strengthens the immune system, the miraculous birth process, healing and recovering from labour."

The Yogic Practise Schedule

a. *First Trimester: The Asanas:*
   – Shavasana   – Veerasana, Dandasana
   – Katichakrasana   – Tadasana

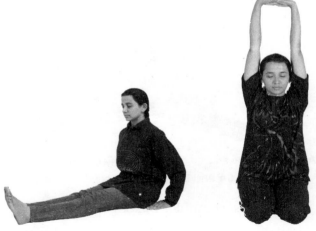

(A) Dandasana   **(B)** Veerasana

Figs 18.5A and B: Asana in first trimester

   – *The Pranayama:* Anulom-vilom breathing and Ujjayi
   breathing.
   – *Dhyana:* Maun dhyana and Mantra dhyana.
The physiotherapy programme as per the regular
schedule.

b. ***Second Trimestor:*** *The Asanas:*
   Standing: Tadasana – the standing pose
               Trikonasana – the triangle pose
   Sitting: Veerasana
               Upvishta konasana
   Lying: Katichakrasana –pelvic rotation to sides

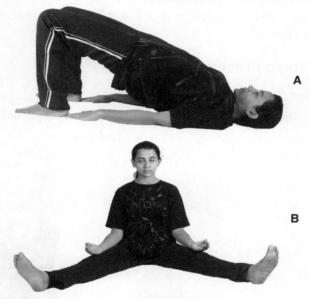

(A) Setubandhasana   **(B)** Modified Upvishtakonasana
Figs 18.6A and B: Asana in second trimestar

   – *The Pranayama:* Anulom vilom breathing
                    Ujjayi breathing.
   – *Dhyana:*   15-20 minutes in any comfortable
                    posture.

c. *Third trimestor:*
  - *The Asanas:*   Tadasana, Baddha konasana, Modified Shavasana, Setubandhasana
  - *The Pranayama:* Anulom vilom breathing Ujjayi breathing
  - *Dhyana:*   15-20 minutes in comfortable sitting position.

"Allow at least eight hours of difference between the Aerobic conditioning physiotherapy sessions and Yogic practise. The Yogic practise is preffered in the morning, relaxation being the main goal of both the sessions."

Physiotherapy Advice During Pregnancy

1. Avoid ballistic movements, i.e. fast repetitive movements
2. Graded, gradual, slow stretching exercises to be continued in all trimesters.
3. Avoid supine lying position after fourth month but can lie down in modified Shavasana position.
4. Always rise up slowly and through side lying to avoid postural hypotension.
5. Avoid breath holding and tendencies that elicit Valsalva manoeuvre.
6. Drink plenty of water, juices, liquids throughout the pregnancy and there after too.
7. Encourage complete bladder emptying before Yogic practise and do not hold.
8. Rest in between sessions in any comfortable position.
9. Practise all Asanas with breath regulation.
10. Follow the whole session as Psychophysical practise.
11. Eat *sattvic* food that will increase vitality, purity, stamina, health, happiness and cheerfulness.

Postnatal Approach and Care—Yogic Practice

Normal Delivery:
- Continue with both the Pranayama as the medical parameters normalise
- Gradually resume to all relaxation Asanas, even in prone lying (lying on belly).
- Asanas in sitting and standing positions included as per guideline.
- Resume all Asanas after three weeks.
- Focus on Concentration and Meditation techniques more often, immediately from next day of delivery.

Caesarian Delivery: The programme cannot be generalized as it will be planned according to the lady's clinical status. Both the Pranayamas, can be practised along with Concentration and Meditation techniques frequently throughout the day.

3. Menopause

- It is defined as the time at which menstruation in woman ceases.
- This occurs between the ages of 45 and 50 years and the period may vary from 2 to 3 years.
- It is also common that a woman continues to menstruate after 50 years.
- The Hormonal levels variate during this period.
- Neurological symptoms like pins and needles in the extremities are experienced.
- Emotional changes like mental depression and mood swings are common.
- Osteoporosis and musculoskeletal pains are also a common feature.
- BMR may be lowered, hence change in endocrine system function is evident.

- It is during this phase that, the woman needs to be reassured, comforted and cared by all around her with a compassionate attitude.
- The gynaecologist usually advocates Hormonal replacement therapy to take care of the above effects to give the female a feeling of well-being along with their counselling.

"It is during this phase of a woman, that Yogic practise has its best effect, as it takes care of all these dimensions."

The Approach

Table 18.1: Menopause and Integrated approach

The Yogic way...	The physical therapy...
• Asanas like Uttanasana and all forwardbending, all backward bending asanas	• Regular walk, a set of stretching exercise
• Pranayama like Anulom vilom and Ujjayi breathing	• Deep breathing exercises
• Meditation 15-20 minutes session	• Positive communication
• Diet: fresh vegetarian food with seasonal fruits and salads	• Sensible eating and moderation in dietary intake
• Attitude: keep everyone happy	• Be always happy
• Feeling of Healing	• Feeling of care and compassion

4. Gynaec Conditions

(a) Uterine Prolapse

- It is a common complaint, seen in women of menopausal age due to pelvic floor muscle weakness and ligamentous laxity.
- The prolapse could be of different grades as per the severity of weakness and laxity.
- This is associated usually with low back ache and perineal muscles weakness.
- Emotional changes like feeling of embarrassment, fear, insecurity, low esteem, etc. are very common in female during this stage.

"Regular Yogic practise, awareness and motivation to woman can help in preventing this agonising problem and proper supervision and guidence can help her in overcoming it too."

Approach

Table 18.2: Uterine prolapse and integrated approach

The Yogic way	The Physical therapy
• Asana like: - Uttanasana - Sarvangasana - Upvista konasana - Padhastasana	• Kegel's exercise programme for pelvic floor muscle strengthening.
• Asanas strengthen pelvic floor and abdominal muscles both	• Abdominal muscles strengthening
• Pranayama: - Anulom vilom - Ujjayi breathing	• Deep breathing exercises
• Bandh (Abdominal lock)	• Isometric abdominal exercise
• Meditation 15-20 minutes daily	• Progressive muscular relaxation

(b) Stress Incontinence

- Incontinence is the difficulty that the woman experiences to control urine at will.
- It is an extremely common symptom in woman with multiple deliveries, and above 40 years of age.
- There is a very small quantity of urine loss whenever there is rise in intra-abdominal pressure during laughing, coughing, lifting, running or even fast walking.
- The psychological importance of stress incontinence should never be underestimated.
- Sometimes psychogenic obesity also precipitates the cause.
- Genuine stress incontinence is due to incompetent urinary sphincter.
- Post menopausal atrophy is also the cause in some.
- In some women it may purely be a Functional Disorder due to Psychological factors.

"It is in this aspect and phase, that the Yogic practise takes care of this problem in a woman."

The Approach

Table 18.3: Stress incontinence and integrated approach

The Yogic way...	The Physical therapy...
Asanas: Veerasana Sarvangasana Baddhakonasana Pranayama: • Anulom vilom • Ujjayi breath Meditation: 15 to 20 minutes daily.	• Kegel's exercise programme for pelvic floor muscles training • Deep breathing exercises for physical relaxation • Relaxation training for mental relaxation.

PRECAUTIONS WHILE DOING ASANAS

All Asanas have a psychophysical purpose with breath regulation and mental relaxation hence the detrimental effects are minimal, but it is necessary to take precautions in all situations and at all levels as the ultimate aim of Yogic practise is Energy Conservation.

1. *Low Back Pain:* • All Asanas are indicated but avoid *Uttanpadasana* (bilateral SLR).

2. *Extreme Fatigue:* • Concentrate on Pranayama. Anulom vilom in any comfortable sitting position.
   • Meditation 15-20 minutes daily replenishes and rejuvenates oneself.

3. *Anaemia:* • Practice regularly pranayama, Anulom-vilom and Ujjayi
   • Diet care.

4. *Phlebitis:* • *Pranayama,* Anulom-vilom and Ujjayi has amazing benefit.

5. *Infections:* • All relaxation Asanas and both the Pranayamas.

6. *Diastesis Rectii:* • It is separation of rectus abdominis muscle in the midline of abdominal wall (lower) which disturbs the continuity of abdominal wall.

Self examination: • If separation is two finger width at umbilicus.
   • Asana to avoid: Uttanpadason (bilateral SLR) and Sarvangasana.
   • Asanas beneficial are Setubandh-asana (Bridging). Pawanmuktasana, Uttan-asana, Utkat-asana and Paschimottan-asana.

CONTRAINDICATION TO ANY YOGASANA PRACTISE

• Incompetent cervix
• Vaginal bleeding
• Maternal heart disease and maternal diabetes
• Intrauterine growth

In all the above conditions, the yogic practice that can be followed include.

The Relaxation Asanas should be focused upon in any condition without stress.

Pranayama: Anulom vilom which is called as "Nadi Shodhan"— the cleansing breathing technique for all channels of body should be practised in any condition.

Meditation 20-30 minutes daily has healing effect mentally and physically.

SUMMARY

1. Asanas aims are to train the mind and body for spiritual perfection and not mere physical exercise.
2. Every posture should be given a Spiritual uplift.
3. Asanas fulfill all the aspects for rehabilitation in woman's health.
4. Pranayama adds meaning to life of a woman and replenishes and recharges her for different roles to perform.
5. Meditation practise brings in her life peace and harmony and prevents her from falling into stressful situations.

"This specialised area of treatment in woman's health is enjoying great growth within physical therapy."

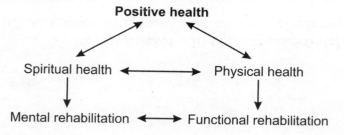

A person's illness or dysfunction is related to how the individual measures himself or herself to the limitation of the physical symtoms. If the person's focus is on deficiencies rather than, on assets, the extent of illness will increase. (Power of mind). Hence, if positive inputs, self prescription techniques and approaches (Yoga) are encouraged to any person, acceptance levels and stress coping mechanism is strengthened.

The reaction one makes to any illness or loss of function is an adjustment process that contributes to one's physical symptoms. If positive emotions are nurtured at all levels of therapies by training and healing the mind, the physical adjustment also becomes easy and acceptable and thus enhance this complete rehabilitation programme of an individual.

EACH AND EVERY INDIVIDUAL IS UNIQUE

Each and every individual's interaction with the internal and external reality is selective and subjective. Catering to these biological, psychological and social needs, require the balancing of internal and external resources.

Living is a constantly ongoing adjustment and adaptation process, encompassing different levels of role demands **physical, mental, social and spiritual**. All these four aspects should be viewed as part of adjustment in general and cannot be viewed as separate entity.

The physical and social aspects of living are external reality demands (*Yama, Niyama, Asana*) whereas the mental and spiritual aspects are internal supply system (*Pratyahara, Dharna, Dhyana*). The balance between the demand (body) and supply (mind) is Pranayama. By gaining control over life force-The Prana- the Breath, one can attain perfect health for physical, mental, social and spiritual aspect of rehabilitation.

"Yoga helps in improving adaptation at physical, psychological physiological and social level of one's functioning."

THE SPIRITUAL QUOTIENT "SELF"

It is the foundation of total health. When the Intelligent Quotient (mind) and Moral Quotient (values) of a healer gets tuned with the Emotional Quotient (subconscious mind functioning) of patient, the results of it speaks for itself.

A heart full of love (*Bhakti yoga*) a mind full of vision (*Gyan yoga*) and hands full of skill (*Karma yoga*) is the true nature of the healer.

Obstacles to inculcate Spiritual quotient and Complete health are disease, laziness, doubt, fatigue (mind and body), desires, ignorance, expectations, fear, grief and sorrow.

Means to remove these obstacles and achieve Complete health are sense withdrawal (Pratyahara), breath regulation (Pranayama), Meditation (Dhyana) and last but most important means is "regular practice" of these with dedication, determination and devotion.

"When applying the principles of Ashtangyoga for disease prevention and cure, the effort is not to prove but is to share my experience of my learning and experiencing of this healing therapy."

THE POWER OF "SELF" IN REHABILITATION

More important than physical cleansing is cleansing of the mind. Physical stability and harmony is a result of quiet, calm serene mind and a regulated breath.

Exercise with its psychophysical concept when practised, regularly and with a purpose or replenishing the energy stores, rehabilitates a person mentally, physically, socially and spiritually - (the missing dimension in today's approach).

Disease cannot be cured completely but emotions can be calmed down. Yoga unveils the curtain of ignorance and makes ones thoughts and actions more flexible and accommodative, thereby aiding mental and muscular relaxation at all levels of functioning.

For rehabilitation, may it be for Cardiovascular conditions, Respiratory conditions, Musculoskeletal conditions, Neurological conditions or Gynaecological conditions, more than exercise, it is the patient's education that is important. The "self prescription and management skills-Yoga" takes care of a "Human being".

The Integraged Approach of Physical therapy (body) and Yoga (mind and soul) will take care of both, the nature (physique) and nurturing element (mind) of the body and rehabilitate a person in all aspects of adaptation, leading to Positive Health (Physical, Mental, Social and Spiritual).

Yoga is not a subtiture for any therapy, modality or clinical skill but it can enable a more integrated approach in rehabilitation.

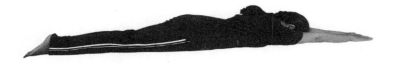

Fig. 19.1: Samarpanasana—Complete surrender to God

This specialized area of approach in health is also enjoying a great growth within medical care and rehabilitation.

Skill in Hands
Vision in Mind
Love in Heart
And
Surrender to God
is true nature of and for rehabilitation

List of Figure and Table Numbers

Figure Nos.

Table Nos.

Index